Michael Wand

Advancing Electromyographic Continuous Speech Recognition

Signal Preprocessing and Modeling

Advancing Electromyographic Continuous Speech Recognition

Signal Preprocessing and Modeling

by
Michael Wand

KIT Scientific Publishing

Dissertation, Karlsruher Institut für Technologie (KIT)
Fakultät für Informatik
Tag der mündlichen Prüfung: 14. Januar 2014
Referenten: Prof. Dr.-Ing. Tanja Schultz, Prof. Philip Green, PhD

Impressum

KIT Scientific Publishing

Karlsruher Institut für Technologie (KIT)
KIT Scientific Publishing
Straße am Forum 2
D-76131 Karlsruhe

KIT Scientific Publishing is a registered trademark of Karlsruhe Institute of Technology. Reprint using the book cover is not allowed.

www.ksp.kit.edu

Print on Demand 2014

ISBN 978-3-7315-0211-1
DOI 10.5445/KSP/1000040667

Advancing Electromyographic Continuous Speech Recognition: Signal Preprocessing and Modeling

Zur Erlangung des akademischen Grades eines
Doktors der Ingenieurwissenschaften
von der Fakultät für Informatik
des Karlsruher Instituts für Technologie (KIT)

genehmigte

Dissertation

von

Michael Wand
aus Göttingen

Tag der mündlichen Prüfung:	14. 1. 2014
Erster Gutachter:	Prof. Dr.-Ing. Tanja Schultz
Zweiter Gutachter:	Prof. Philip Green, PhD

Summary

Speech is the most natural medium of communication between humans, and an increasingly important tool to control technical devices. Therefore speech is of tremendous significance to every human being, and to society as a whole.

However, speech must normally be pronounced in a clearly audible manner, particularly if it is to be transmitted via a technical device, for example a cellphone, or processed e.g. by a speech recognizer. This is problematic in a number of situations: First, when a person communicates via spoken speech, the environment may be disturbed. This happens in public places, for example libraries or restaurants, as well as in meetings or open-plan offices. Second, confidential communication is impossible: PINs or passwords, which are frequently needed to gain access to a voice-controlled computer system, are particularly endangered. Third, speech-disabled persons may be excluded from both interaction with other humans and using speech-controlled devices.

Therefore the development of alternative methods of capturing and processing speech is becoming increasingly popular. Our method of choice is Silent Speech recognition by surface electromyography (EMG), where the electrical potentials of a user's articulatory muscles are captured by surface electrodes attached to the face: This makes it possible to capture and process speech even if *no acoustic signal is produced, or can be measured* (the latter may be interesting in places with high background noise).

This thesis aims at enhancing and improving myoelectric Silent Speech recognition. Based on a standard speech recognition toolchain, we systematically develop methods and algorithms to adapt these components in a way specifically suited for the EMG signal. While our main goal is to improve the recognition accuracy of the Silent Speech recognizer, we also include analyses at the signal and model level, so that we gain a better understanding of the system. Our baseline is an EMG-based speech recognizer which was state-of-the-art at the beginning of our research, we show that we can substantially improve its power, flexibility, and robustness.

The main achievements of this thesis are as follows:

EMG Signal Capture and Processing The myoelectric signal is a complex superposition of signals from many different sources (muscles and muscle fibers). Therefore we introduce an EMG recording system based on *electrode arrays*, which are grid structures with multiple EMG measuring points, and show that we can use the resulting high-dimensional signal to gain information about these sources which is not available in classical recording systems. The first concrete application is an artifact removal algorithm using source separation techniques.

Flexible myoelectric modeling We observed during our experiments that standard phone models, which are used in conventional speech recognition, are not well suited for our system, particularly not when only a small amount of training data is available. We introduce *Phonetic Feature Bundling*, a robust and powerful alternative to phone modeling which yields a remarkable Word Error Rate reduction of up to 40.8% relative.

Analysis and enhancement of silently mouthed speech It is well-known that silently mouthed speech exhibits properties different from normal ("audible") speech. This causes accuracy degradation when a system is applied across different *speaking modes*. An analysis of silent speech at the signal level leads us to the development of a signal-based adaptation method which ameliorates this problem and improves the recognition of silent speech.

Session independency and adaptation The myoelectric signal changes when the electrodes are removed and reattached between recording sessions. Clearly this is a major issue in practical usage scenarios. We show that *session-independent* systems are possible, so that an enrollment immediately before usage is no longer necessary. In addition, adaptation can be used to further improve such a system; we show in particular that *unsupervised adaptation* is possible: EMG data can be accrued during usage of the system and be used for improving the recognizer. This is a major step forward since such data is available in far larger amounts than supervised training data, whose generation requires that a user invests time and care.

Online demonstration system We present an online, real-time demonstration system which makes use of most of the methods developed in this thesis. This proves our concepts to have an immediate practical impact, and shows the potential of applied EMG-based speech recognition.

Zusammenfassung

Sprache ist das natürlichste zwischenmenschliche Kommunikationsmedium und darüberhinaus für die Steuerung von technischen Geräten zunehmend wichtig. Daher hat Sprache eine enorme Bedeutung, sowohl für jeden einzelnen Menschen als auch für die Gesellschaft insgesamt.

Sprache muss normalerweise klar hörbar sein, besonders dann, wenn eine maschinelle Verarbeitung (z.B. durch einen Spracherkenner) oder Übertragung (etwa mittels mobiler Telefonie) erwünscht ist. Dies ist unter mehreren Aspekten problematisch: Erstens beeinträchtigt laute Sprachkommunikation die Umgebung. Dies kann öffentliche Orte betreffen, wie Bibliotheken oder Restaurants, aber kann auch in Besprechungen oder im Großraumbüro ein Problem sein. Zweitens ist vertrauliche Kommunikation unmöglich: Gerade PINs oder Passwörter, die man beispielsweise zum Zugriff auf ein sprachbasiertes Interaktionssystem übermitteln möchte, sind gefährdet. Drittens sind sprachbehinderte Menschen unter Umständen sowohl von der Kommunikation mit Menschen als auch von der sprachlichen Interaktion mit Maschinen ausgeschlossen.

Daher werden inzwischen verstärkt alternative Sprachkommunikationsformen erforscht. Die in dieser Arbeit verwendete Methode ist Spracherkennung durch Oberflächenelektromyographie (EMG): Die elektrischen Potentiale der Artikulationsmuskeln werden gemessen, indem man Elektroden auf das Gesicht des Sprechers aufbringt. Dadurch wird es möglich, Sprache auch dann zu erfassen und zu verarbeiten, wenn *kein akustisches Signal erzeugt wird oder messbar ist* (der zweite Aspekt ist zum Beispiel bei starken Hintergrundgeräuschen interessant).

Diese Arbeit befasst sich mit der Erweiterung und Verbesserung eines myoelektrischen Spracherkenners. Die Komponenten der in der Spracherkennung üblichen Prozesskette werden systematisch für die EMG-basierte Spracherkennung angepasst, bzw. es werden neue Algorithmen und Methoden entwickelt. Das Hauptziel ist die Verbesserung der Erkennungsgenauigkeit, darüber hinaus erweist es sich als lehrreich, Analysen des Signals und der Erkennermodelle durchzuführen. Ein EMG-basierter Spracherkenner, der zu Beginn dieser Arbeit Stand der Technik war, dient als Grundlage für diese hier vorgestellten Experimente; es wird gezeigt, dass sich Genauigkeit, Flexibilität und Robustheit dieses Erkenners beträchtlich verbessern lassen.

Die Hauptergebnisse der Arbeit lassen sich wie folgt zusammenfassen:

Verarbeitung des EMG-Signals Das myoelektrische Signal ist eine komplexe Überlagerung von Signalen, die aus verschiedenen Quellen (Muskeln und Muskelfasern) stammen. Daher wurde ein Aufnahmesystem entwickelt, das auf *Elektrodenarrays* – Gitterstrukturen mit regelmäßig angeordneten EMG-Messpunkten – basiert und es ermöglicht, Informationen über diese Quellen zu extrahieren, die man mit klassischen Aufnahmesystemen nicht erhalten kann. Die erste konkrete Anwendung dieses Systems ist ein Artefaktbereinigungsalgorithmus, der auf Quellenseparation basiert.

Flexible myoelektrische Modellierung Es zeigte sich im Verlauf dieser Arbeit, dass phon-basierte Modellierung, die in der konventionellen Spracherkennung verwendet wird, nicht gut für das hier vorgestellte System geeignet ist, besonders dann nicht, wenn nur sehr wenig Trainingsdaten verfügbar sind. Es wird *Phonetic Feature Bundling* als robuste und leistungsfähige alternative Modellierungsform eingeführt und gezeigt, dass damit Verbesserungen der Wortfehlerrate von bis zu 40.8% relativ erreicht werden.

Analyse und Verbesserung lautloser Sprache Es ist bekannt, dass sich die Eigenschaften lautlos artikulierter und normal gesprochener Sprache unterscheiden. Dies verringert die Erkennungsgenauigkeit eines Systems, das über *Sprachmodi* hinweg angewendet wird. Eine Analyse der EMG-Signale liefert die Grundlage zur Entwicklung einer signalbasierten Adaptionsmethode, die den Unterschied zwischen den EMG-Signalen normaler und lautloser Sprache verringert und somit die Wortfehlerrate verbessert.

Sitzungsunabhängigkeit und Adaption Das EMG-Signal verändert sich, wenn zwischen Aufnahme*sitzungen* die EMG-Elektroden entfernt und neu angebracht werden – dies ist ein bedeutendes Problem in praktischen Anwendungsszenarien. In dieser Arbeit wird gezeigt, dass *sitzungsunabhängige* Systeme möglich sind. Damit ist ein Training des Systems direkt vor der Anwendung nicht mehr nötig, zusätzlich kann ein sitzungsunabhängiges System durch Adaptionsmethoden verbessert werden. Insbesondere wird gezeigt, dass *unüberwachte* Adaption möglich ist: Daten können während der Benutzung des Systems gesammelt und zur Verbesserung der Erkennungsleistung verwendet werden. Dies ist ein bedeutender Fortschritt, weil solche Daten in weit größerer Menge als überwachte Trainingsdaten verfügbar sind; um letztere zu erhalten, ist ein gewisser Zeitaufwand vom Benutzer erforderlich.

Online-Demonstrationssystem Es wird ein echtzeitfähiges Demonstrationssystem präsentiert, das mehrere der in dieser Arbeit entwickelten Methoden verwendet. Dies beweist, dass die hier vorgestellten Konzepte eine unmittelbare praktische Bedeutung haben, und zeigt das Potential der angewandten EMG-basierten Spracherkennung.

Acknowledgements

A dissertation is never the work of a single person, but only becomes possible by the help and collaboration of many people. This includes students, colleagues, and fellow scientists, who have influenced and assisted my studies in various ways, and my friends and my family, who always supported and encouraged me.

First of all, I wish to thank Prof. Tanja Schultz, my primary supervisor and head of Cognitive Systems Lab (CSL) at Karlsruhe Institute of Technology. With her incessant enthusiasm, she aroused my interest in both speech recognition and biosignal processing, and during my work, she supported me with a multitude of ideas, encouraging and empowering me to pursue my own directions of study. I also emphasize the assistance I received in building my scientific network: This study would not be the same without the stimulations I got from diverse conferences, meetings, and discussions with other researchers.

The latter turned out to be particularly important since I made my way into somewhat "uncharted territory", with only a small community of fellow investigators working on the topic of Silent Speech recognition. One of them is highly respected Prof. Philip Green, who I thank for enlightening discussions during a visit in Sheffield and on various conferences, and particularly for co-supervising my thesis and giving highly useful remarks on the final written version.

My colleagues in Karlsruhe, as well as several of the highly capable students who I supervised, have not only greatly supported my work, but also have become friends. My colleagues were, in order of office room numbers: Dirk Gehrig, Christoph Amma, Felix Putze, Dominic Heger, Christian Herff, Matthias Janke, Tim Schlippe, Thang Vu, and Dominic Telaar. Very particularly, I wish to thank Matthias for a long collaboration on EMG-based Silent Speech interfaces during the course of several years. Marcus Georgi and Jochen Weiner recently joined the ranks of CSL researchers.

Present and past student members of the EMG team include, but are not limited to, Cindy Dettmann, Lorenz Diener, Till Heistermann, Adam Himmelsbach, Michael Ikkert, Christopher Schulte, and Marlene Zahner. Some of them are co-authors of my papers, or contributed to this dissertation by writing their own

Diploma/Bachelor/Master theses, others assisted in programming or recording tasks. They all formed a close-knit team and often worked far more than I could decently ask of them. I hope that the support Matthias and I gave them as co-supervisors and team leaders helps them to find their place in science (preferrably, but anywhere else in life would also be OK), if this happens, our work was not in vain.

I received very important support from Szu-Chen Jou from Carnegie Mellon University, my "predecessor" in Silent Speech research, and my co-advisor when I first started a student research project on speech recognition using biosignals, back in 2006. He greatly helped me to get started, and a large part of my initial codebase was originally his. Alfred Schmidt became our system administrator towards the end of my time at CSL, and all the sudden, things which used to take up a lot of our scarce time worked flawlessly. Helga Scherer, our secretary, never lost track of anything related to administration of budgets, travels, teaching, or research, and she always knew whom to ask for a problem solution. She greatly aided me during my time at CSL.

My parents, Gudrun and Gerhard Wand, constantly encouraged and supported me, and I extend my warmest thanks to them. Many friends have accompanied me during my time in Karlsruhe (and before), and I would like to add their names here. However, in order to keep the complexity of this section under control, I refrain from actually writing out this list, and I am sure that any of my friends who reads this section knows that he or she is addressed.

Contents

List of Figures

List of Tables

Chapter 1

Introduction and Motivation

This chapter serves as a motivation for the present dissertation, and as an introduction to the field. We introduce spoken language as a cornerstone of human communication, motivate the development of Silent Speech Interfaces, and give an overview of existing techniques. Finally, the structure and contributions of this thesis are presented.

1.1 Speech as an Ubiquitous Means of Communication

It is widely accepted that spoken communication is a key capability of human beings. Certainly, speech is the most complex form of communication which is known to us, and its importance cannot be underestimated: In our daily lives, speech is used for efficient transmission of vital information, for the organization of life in a complex, multi-faceted society, for communicating desires and intentions, and for social interaction, just to name a few examples.

However, it requires relatively complex technology to store or transmit spoken language. This makes speech a very volatile form of communication: all but 150 years ago, spoken communication was limited to personal conversation or speeches in front of at most medium-sized audiences, bound to the present and bound to a specific location. Speech and language could only be conserved in written form, in chronicles, books, or letters.

We argue that speech has evolved drastically since this time: The telephone, first patented in 1876 by Alexander Graham Bell, allowed for the first time to talk to persons at distant locations [Bro94]. Just one year later, in 1877, Thomas Edison invented the "phonograph", the first device ever which could record and playback arbitrary sounds [Str]. These developments are among the most famous in a series of groundbreaking inventions which took place during the last two centuries: they drastically changed our society and, concerning the topic of this thesis, affected the use of speech, which is now used for more and more purposes.

In which ways is speech being used nowadays? During the past decades, the evolution of speech-based communication has even increased its pace. Mobile phones became widely available around 25 years ago and have gained enormous popularity since then, making speech communication ubiquitous: Instantaneous spoken communication with any person, anywhere on the world, has become a reality. A further purpose of speech which has emerged during the past decades is operating technical devices: speech-driven programs and appliances range from telephone-based customer service dispatch and voice-controlled personal assistants, which normally recognize a small set of words, to large-vocabulary dictation and translation systems which recognize and process fluent ("continuous") speech.

1.2 Introducing Silent Speech Interfaces

In the last paragraph we justified the assertion that speech-based mobile communication and speech-controlled human-computer interaction have become ubiquitous technologies with enormous practical importance. However they induce several specific problems [DSH+10, SW10]: First, acoustic speech signals are transmitted through air and are thus susceptible to environmental noise. Therefore speech recognizers degrade quite drastically when they are used in places like crowded restaurants, airports, etc. Also cellphone-based communication is severely hindered.

Second, speech needs to be clearly audible, particularly when it is to be transmitted or processed by technical systems. In quiet places, like libraries, meetings, etc., this disturbs bystanders, making this means of communication unsuitable in a variety of situations.

Third, private spoken communication is vulnerable: There is a real danger of being overheard. This is undesired or embarrassing at best and dangerous at worst, when confidential information is to be transmitted. Speech-controlled services which require PINs, passwords, or security information are particularly affected.

Fourth, speech-disabled people may be excluded both from speech-based communication with other persons and from speech-driven human-machine interaction. There exists a variety of reasons why a person might be unable to speak, the most severe of them is a paralysis of the full body, the so-called *locked-in* syndrome. For the purpose of this thesis, we consider cases where the articulatory muscles still function normally, but a voice may not be produced; such a situation is typical for *laryngectomy* patients, where the vocal chords have been removed.

Silent Speech Interface (SSI) technology allows to utter speech silently and thus provides a way to solve the problems described above: confidential information can be submitted securely, silent speech does not disturb or interfere with the surroundings, and it is possible to create speech prostheses for speech-disabled patients.

Modern sensor technology provides the means to construct a variety of Silent Speech interfaces, for an overview of current research see section 1.3. Our approach to capture speech without using the acoustic signal uses surface ElectroMyoGraphy (EMG) [Kra07, Chapter 11], which is the process of recording electrical muscle activity using surface electrodes. Since speech is produced by the activity of the human articulatory muscles, the myoelectric signal patterns captured from a person's face allow to trace back the corresponding speech. Since EMG relies on muscle activity only, speech can be recognized even when it is produced silently, i.e. mouthed without any vocal effort. In section 1.4 the state-of-the-art of EMG-based speech processing is presented; a summary of background knowledge regarding the origin and measurement of the EMG signal is found in section 2.1.

1.3 Silent Speech Processing Technologies

Research in the field of Silent Speech Interfaces (SSI) has got several decades of history. In the following an overview of available technologies is given, based on the excellent summary article [DSH+10]. EMG-based approaches are of particular interest to us, they are considered in detail in section 1.4.

According to [DSH+10], the "first 'true' SSI system, although with very limited performance", was based on electromyography: In 1985, Sugie and Tsunoda devised a recognition system which could discriminate five Japanese vowels, capturing facial EMG with three sensors [ST85]. The system used signals from 3

EMG channels, captured from the speaker's face, for recognition of 5 Japanese vowels. A different method was presented in 1992: Hasegawa and colleagues proposed a "lipreading" system driven by camera images of the lips, also performing phone recognition [HO92].

Since these early beginnings, the variety of Silent Speech processing systems has increased a lot. The technologies may be grouped into three categories:

- Capture of very quiet speech signals. This may be done by bone conduction, stethoscopic microphones, etc., and requires that at least a small sound is produced. Nonetheless, these technologies address the same problems as true *silent* speech interfaces and are therefore considered in this summary.
- Capture of vocal tract or articulator configurations, e.g. by electromyography, or by visual or ultrasound imaging. This allows to recognize speech even when no sound is produced and is our method of choice.
- Direct interpretation of brain signals related to speech production. This is by far the most complicated method due to the complexity of the human brain activity.

Each of these methods has advantages and drawbacks, and some of them might not be suitable for all possible tasks in Silent Speech recognition. In the following, a detailed list is given.

The following acoustics-based approaches, i.e. approaches that capture a (quiet) acoustic signal, exist:

- Acoustic speech recording with a stethoscopic microphone is a well-researched and promising method [NKCS06, HKSS07]. Here, acoustic signals are conducted via the body and are captured with a stethoscope-like microphone originally invented by Nakajima and colleagues [NKSC03]. Due to the high sensitivity of this technology, the system can process almost inaudible speech sounds, for which Nakajima coined the term "Non-audible murmur" (NAM).
- A special application of stethoscopic microphones in the field of speech protheses is the capture of speech signals generated by an electrolarynx. Such devices are used for persons who lack vocal folds (typically as a result of cancer), they generate an artificial vocal excitation so that speaking becomes possible, but the resulting speech is known to be very unnatural [MH05b]. However, it has been shown that with the NAM technology, it is possibly to capture very quiet electrolaryngeal speech, which is unhearable for bystanders. This signal can then be processed to make the resulting speech more natural [HOS+10, TBLT10, NTSS12].

- Acoustic activity may be captured using electromagnetic sensors (electroglottography) [TSB+00, NBHG00, Tar03, PFC06, QBM+06] or vibration sensors [BT05, PH10]. Like NAM, these methods rely on speech signals transmitted via the human body, so they require that some kind of acoustic signal is produced.

The common property of these approaches is their use of the body as a medium for sound signal conduction, thus avoiding the aforementioned inherent problems of standard audio recording by microphones, and enabling the capture of *almost* silent speech signals. Since we consider whispering as a form of covert communication, the above list is to be extended with a last technique: Whispered speech can, of course, also be captured by standard microphones for subsequent recognition [ITI05, JSW05] or enhancement [SMA09].

Still, in certain situations, even a very quiet acoustic signal might be unavailable or undesired, or it might be lacking in quality or naturalness. In such cases, different speech capturing methods are required. The following approaches record activity of the vocal tract, i.e. of the articulators. It is expected that such information is sufficient in order to completely retrace the corresponding speech, yet it may be difficult to obtain a full representation of the vocal tract activity (for example, video-based methods might capture the lip position, but fail to yield information about the tongue).

- A silent speech interface based on ultrasound (US) imaging of the vocal tract was first proposed by Denby and colleagues in 2004 [DS04]. As in [HO92], optical capture of the lip movement can additionally be used. During the past 10 years, a substantial amount of research on this method has been performed (see e.g. [DODS06, HAC+07, HBC+10, FCBD+10]). Most image-based systems are limited to the recognition of whole words, i.e. the input data features are compared with templates of the words to be recognized. Recent papers, e.g. [HBD12], tackle the problem of processing continuous speech by using a *direct mapping* between image features and acoustics, bypassing the recognition phase. Classical systems are quite impractical, since the user's head has to be mounted on a fixation device, however portable systems are just underway [DCH+11].
- Exact measurements of articulator activity are created by *Electromagnetic Articulography* (EMA) [SGW+87, HFB+06]. For EMA measurements, small electrical coils are glued to the subject's articulators. A magnetic field is generated outside the human body, and an electrical current is induced in the coils. Small cables connect the coils to a recording apparatus, which captures the generated signal, from which the exact positioning of the articulators may be obtained. To the best of our knowledge, full EMA-based

Silent Speech Interfaces have not yet been reported, however EMA has been used for giving feedback to patients with speech disorders [KBC99] and for acoustic-articulatory inversion, i.e. for computing articulator information from acoustic signals for use in speech recognition and synthesis [UMRR12]. The main drawback of the EMA technology is its invasiveness, in particular, electrical coils need to be glued to the subjects lips, tongue, etc., and the coils need to have a cable connection to a recording device.

- Despite the invasiveness of EMA, directly tracking the activity of the articulators is highly desirable. In 2008, Fagan and colleagues [FEG+08] proposed to replace the coils by very small permanent magnets, which cause almost no discomfort for the user and might in the future even be implanted. The activity of the magnets is then measured outside the human body, and the resulting signal can be used for a Silent Speech Interface [HEF+10, GRH+10, HEF+13, HBC+13]. This very promising technique has been named "Permanent-magnetic articulography" (PMA), a particular advantage is its mobility: Recent systems are fully portable, thus potentially allowing usage in everyday situations in the near future.
- Electromyography (EMG) has been used for some of the earliest non-acoustic speech processing systems [ST85, MDTM89]. Here the electrical activity of the articulatory muscles is captured with electrodes, see section 2.1 for details. In section 1.4, we review the research on EMG-based speech processing.

Finally, it should be possible to capture speech information at its source, namely, at the human brain. Many difficulties arise from any such approach, since accurately measuring brain activity is a challenging task. Electroencephalography, where the electrical activity of the cortex is measured with surface electrodes attached to the user's head, is a straightforward and relatively cost-effective approach, unfortunately it only yields a very crude and incomplete image of the brain activity. In particular, it is very hard to determine the exact source position of a signal, so it is all but impossible to directly recognize activity patterns related to different articulators. Imaging methods, like fMRI, are usually not considered for this task since their time resolution is too low: It is known that during normal speech, around 10-30 phones per second are generated, so any recording method would have to capture at least 10-30 samples per second. This is a far higher recording frequency than standard imaging systems are *currently* able to achieve, the typical amount of time required for a full brain scan ranges around 2-3 seconds. Yet, faster systems are under way, for example, [FMS+10] reports the development of an fMRI method allowing to capture multiple images per second.

Nonetheless, brain signals are used for communication and control. *Brain computer interfaces* are intended to enable communication for severely disabled patients [DdRMH+07]. Usually, they allow the discrimination of a small number of classes of brain activity, they are not normally speech-based. The following methods of brain activity based Silent Speech recognition have been investigated:

- Isolated word recognition by surface electroencephalography was investigated in [SLH97, Wes06, PWCS09]. Notably, widely varying recognition rates were observed, depending on the subject and the setup.
- Interpretation of signals from electrodes implanted into the speech-motor cortex brain area was investigated by Brumberg et al. [BNCKG10]. Of course, this is a highly invasive technology which is only suitable for severely disabled patients for whom no other means of communication remains.

No brain signal based Silent Speech interface even comes close to achieving continuous speech recognition based on smaller units than words. Therefore, from the standpoint of applicability, investigating the second class of Silent Speech interfaces, where articulatory activity is measured, is most promising. Here the EMG approach compares favorably in terms of usability, power, non-invasiveness, and cost [DSH+10].

1.4 Related Work in Myoelectric Speech Recognition

As reported above, research on EMG-based speech recognition began with the works of Sugie et al. [ST85] and Morse et al. [MDTM89]. The early systems exhibited rather low performance. Competitive results were first reported in 2001 by Chan and colleagues [CEHL01], reaching an average word accuracy of 93% on a 10-word vocabulary consisting of the English digits. A good performance could be achieved even when words were spoken non-audibly, i.e. when no acoustic signal was produced [JLA03], paving the way towards a true Silent Speech interface.

The following years saw few progress, until renewed interest in Silent Speech interfaces, possibly due to the increasing use of cellphones, spurred further research in EMG-based speech recognition [DSH+10]. In 2005, L. Maier-Hein conducted a sizable study on optimal parameters and setups for an EMG-based speech recognition system based on the *Varioport* biosignal recorder, one of the first mobile devices of its kind. The results of these experiments were mostly laid down in Maier-Hein's diploma thesis [MH05a] and in the subsequent publication [MHMSW05]. The optimal setup from that study is still in use and was applied for the majority of experiments in this thesis, it is described in section 3.1.1; only recently, we developed a new data recording setup based on multi-channel *EMG arrays*, see section 3.1.2 and chapter 7.

The introduction of phone models to EMG-based speech recognition, achieved in 2006 by S. Jou [JSW+06], can be considered as the next major stepping stone towards a practically useful system. Before this result, EMG-based speech recognizers worked on a whole-word basis, comparing a word to be recognized with a template. This limits the recognizer vocabulary to just a few words, since for each word which might possibly be recognized, training examples must be recorded. Phone-based modeling allows to assemble models for whole words out of the constituting phones (speech sounds), as described in section 2.3.2. This enables potentially unlimited vocabularies as well as data sharing and reuse, among other benefits. Syllable-based recognition, being a compromise between unflexible whole-word units and small phone units, has also been considered [WKJ+06, LLMAM10]. The experiments presented in this thesis start from the recognition system devised in [JSW+06], including some modifications which have been reported in [JSW07].

Beyond the scope of this thesis, further research topics in EMG-based speech processing include

- optimized feature extraction for single-electrode systems [MCDH11], in this study novel signal preprocessing methods are investigated in the context of the EMG array setup
- the application of electromyography in special circumstances, e.g. for firefighters and special forces who may be prevented from speaking because they wear a breathing apparatus [JD10],
- recognition of *disordered speech*, i.e. speech produced by disabled persons [DPH+09]
- language-dependent challenges, e.g. nasality detection [FTD12]
- direct synthesis of speech from EMG signals [TWS09, Lee10, NJWS11, JWNS12], which among other advantages allows modeling prosodic information [JJWS12].

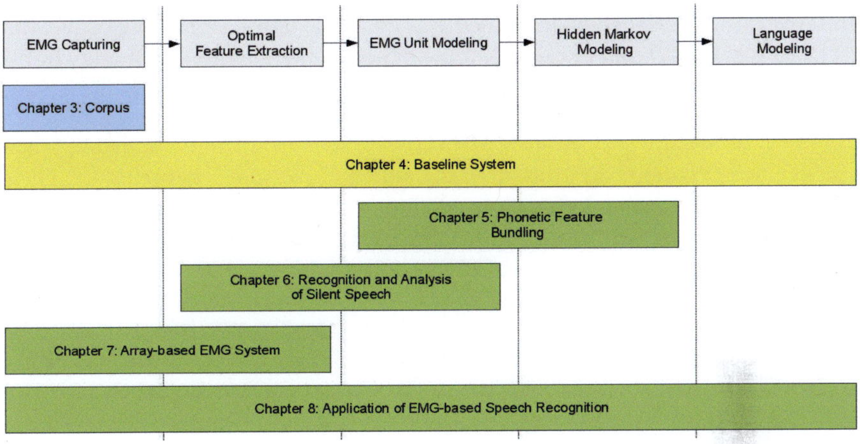

Figure 1.1 – Structure of the experiments and results presented in this thesis

1.5 Structure and Contributions of this Work

This thesis is structured as follows. The first part consists of chapters 1 and 2 and introduces the reader to the purpose of this thesis, to the required background, and to related work in both EMG-based speech recognition and other types of Silent Speech interfaces. The main part consists of chapters 3 to 8 and presents the experimental setup, the baseline recognizer which serves as a starting point for this study, and the key results. Chapter 9 concludes the thesis.

Since this thesis aims at investigating, analysing, and improving all parts of the EMG speech recognition processing chain, the main part is rather large and comprehensive. In order to obtain a structured approach, the results are arranged in relation to this processing chain.

This concept is depicted in figure 1.1. The top row shows the main building blocks of the recognizer, i.e. signal capturing, feature extraction, unit modeling, Hidden Markov models as an instance of sequence modeling, and finally, language modeling. The nonstandard term *unit modeling* is used to refer to the modeling of single frames, without considering sequence constraints.

The lower rows each correspond to one chapter of the main part of the thesis and relate it to specific parts of the processing chain. We begin with chapter 3, where the EMG recording setup is introduced and the properties of the corpora are presented. While an established electrode configuration based on a set of single electrodes was taken from earlier studies [MHMSW05], a new setup based on multi-channel EMG *arrays* was developed as part of this thesis. Chapter 4 presents the speech recognizer which was available at the beginning of this thesis [JSW+06, Jou08] and upon which the experiments and improvements in this thesis are built. An analysis of the capabilities of this recognizer is performed, yielding insight into typical properties of the EMG signals of speech.

The key achievements are presented in chapters 5, 6, and 7, covering the entire processing chain (except language modeling, which is not specific to EMG-based speech recognition and therefore of limited interest in this work). The main contributions of this thesis are as follows:

- Bundled phonetic feature modeling: The specific properties of the EMG data and the small size of the available corpora require an innovative modeling structure. Bundled Phonetic Features combine concepts from context dependent model optimization, modeling of phonetic properties, and information fusion, achieving a Word Error Rate reduction of up to 40.8% relative. See chapter 5.

- Analysis and adaptation for silent speech: The goal of the EMG-based speech recognizer is the recognition of silently mouthed speech, however so far, few investigators considered the discrepancy between silently mouthed and audibly spoken speech. In this thesis a multi-speaker corpus is used to evaluate measures to quantify this discrepancy and to develop a novel signal-based adaptation approach, the *Spectral Mapping* method. Spectral Mapping reduces the Word Error Rates on silent speech by up to 11.5% relative. See chapter 6.

- Electrode Arrays for EMG recording: Previous EMG-based speech recognition systems used a small set of up to around 10 EMG electrodes for signal capture. In this thesis we establish a new recording system based on electrode arrays, which allows the application of advanced signal processing methods; first results are presented on the application of *Independent Component Analysis* for artifact reduction. See chapter 7.

Chapter 8 connects the theoretical results of the thesis with issues of practical application. The following aspects are covered.

- Session independency: It is demonstrated that session-independent and session-adaptive systems are feasible. Session independency means that a user can prepare the system by recording training data at any suitable time, and when he or she needs to apply the system, no further enrollment is necessary. This is a great benefit when EMG-based speech recognition is to be practically applied. We then show that session-independent systems may be further improved by session *adaptation*, in particular, even *unsu-*

pervised adaptation is possible, where data can be accrued during system usage without requiring any particular effort by the user.

- Online demonstration system: A prototype demonstration system using Bundled Phonetic Feature modeling and session adaptation was created. This system has been demonstrated in a variety of settings and situations, including scientific conferences and trade fairs, and was showcased in media and television, including German ZDF and British BBC news.

Chapter 2

Physiological and Technological Background

EMG-based Speech Recognition requires capturing and interpreting a complex biological process. Therefore, the first part of this chapter assembles physiological and technical background information which is required to undertake the task of collecting facial electromyographic signals with the purpose of extracting the underlying speech activity. The second part deals with the physiology of speaking and introduces fundamental concepts regarding the description and classification of speech sounds. In part three we present the building blocks of a classical speech recognition system and introduce methods and terminology which are used in later parts of this thesis. Finally, in part four we describe two important methods for feature dimensionality reduction, namely, Principal Component Analysis and Linear Discriminant Analysis.

2.1 Electromyography – Origin and Capture

2.1.1 Physiology of Human Muscle Contraction

The Musculoskeletal System The outer structure of the human body is determined by the *musculoskeletal system*, i.e. by the joint structure composed of bones, muscles, tendons, ligaments, cartilage, etc. The skeleton supports the different parts of the body and creates a rigid structure, allowing only well-defined movements at specific locations and with limited degrees of freedom. This means that displacements of parts of the body are only possible at the joints, where two

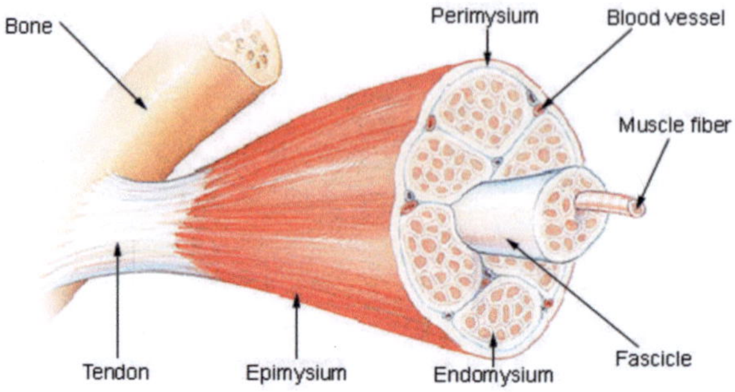

Figure 2.1 – Structure of the human muscle (adapted from [USNIoHb], public domain)

or more bones connect. The possible movements are limited by the structure of the joints and by the supporting ligaments.

Movement of body parts is caused by muscle activity. Muscles can contract, thus pulling parts of the body together, but are unable to exert force by pushing. Therefore, in many cases muscles in the body come in pairs, so that the contraction of one muscle (the *agonist*) has the opposite effect of the contraction of another muscle (the *antagonist*).

Human muscles are subdivided in two categories: *Smooth* musculature, which occurs in inner organs and is not voluntarily controlled, and *striated* musculature, which gains its name from exhibiting a specific periodic structure that is visible under a microscope as a series of stripes. Striated muscles appear as heart muscles and as *skeletal* muscles; the latter are the only muscles in the human body which can be controlled by conscious decisions of the brain. Since speech is produced by conciously moving the articulators, in the following we only consider skeletal muscles.

Figure 2.1 depicts the composition of a typical muscle, here attached to a bone via a *tendon*. The muscle consists of muscle cells, or muscle *fibers*, which mostly comprise *myofibrils*. The myofibrils can change their length, thus causing a contraction of the muscle. In the following the initiation and execution of such a contraction is described.

Properties and Role of Neurons *Neurons* (or nerve cells) are the basic building blocks of the human brain and the nervous system: Thus the functionality of the brain, as well as the transmission of information and control commands between

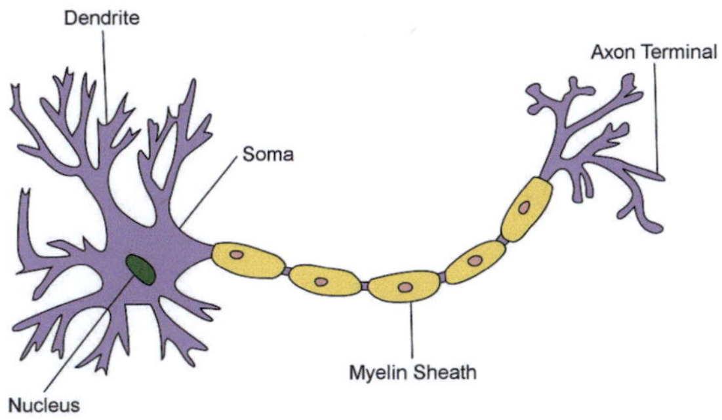

Figure 2.2 – A single neuron. The dendrites collect input signals, the soma performs computations, and the axon conducts the output signal to another cell, e.g. another neuron or a muscle fiber (adapted from [Wik13b], CC-BY-SA-3.0 license).

brain and body, heavily depend on them. Neurons appear in various functions and shapes, but they all share two key properties:

- First, they exhibit a complex, highly branched and interconnected structure. This allows the exchange of information between neurons and the formation of complex neuronal networks, which also connect with other cells of the body. For this thesis, the connection to muscle cells will be of particular interest.
- Second, neurons are able to perform basic computations. While a single neuron is only limitedly powerful, neural networks (far more potent than their computer-simulated counterparts) are able to process complex information. The neural network consisting of the brain and the connected nervous system is the foundation of any (conscious and unconscious) control processes in the human body.

The components of a neuron are shown in figure 2.2: Simply speaking, the *dendrites* collect electrical or chemical input signals. These signals propagate as electrical currents to the *soma*, the bulbous central part of the neuron, where a temporal and spatial summation over the input signals takes place. Finally, the neuron is activated if the voltage in the soma exceeds a certain threshold: An *action potential* forms. This action potential propagates along the *axon*, which thus serves as output conductor for this neuron. The axon connects to other neurons or other cells of the human body.

The shape and life cycle of action potentials is well known [Sch06, Chapter 3–5]: In a non-excited resting state, the neuron exhibits a potential of around -70mV compared to the outside. When the neuron is *depolarized* by incoming stimuli so that its inner potential is greater than approximately -40mV, voltage-triggered ion channels in the cell membrane open, bringing forth an influx of positively charged ions. This causes the inner potential of the neuron to rise to a maximum level of around +30mV, which is independent of the strength of the input excitation ("all-or-nothing principle").

The action potential is a localized depolarization of a part of the axon, traveling away from the soma. Since ion channels exist anywhere on the axon, the action potential sustains itself by further influx of positively charged ions. This makes action potentials suitable for information transport across large distances: indeed, the longest neurons in the human body reach from the spinal cord down to the toes, so their length may exceed one meter [Sch06, Chapter 3]. Within the body, axons are bundled to make signal transport more robust, such a bundle is called a *nerve*.

When a neuron is stimulated continuously, action potentials are repeatedly generated. While all action potentials have identical strength, their frequency carries information about the strength of the excitation. The complex way information is gathered from the dendrites, the all-or-nothing principle, and the frequency encoding of excitation strength makes the activation pattern of a neuron a rather intricate nonlinear process.

Neural Control of Muscle Contraction In general, a voluntary muscle contraction is initiated by a part of the brain called the *motorcortex*. It is part of the outer layer of the brain, i.e. the cortex, where most "high-level" neural processes take place. The motorcortex is located at the center of the head, stretching roughly from ear to ear. Classically, it is assumed that there is a mapping between sections of the motorcortex and the body parts which these sections control [Sch06, Chapter 6], however newer studies indicate that the structure of the motor cortex might be even more complicated [MAKG08].

An activation signal from the motorcortex propagates to a *motoneuron*, which serves as a final point of control for a set of muscle fibers. A motoneuron also processes input signals which cause muscular *reflexes* like the knee-jerk reflex—this means that such reflexes are directly created by the motoneurons, without intervention of the brain. For muscles of the lower body, the controlling motoneuron is located in the spinal cord, for the facial muscles, motoneurons are located within the brain, in specific structures known as *cranial nerve nuclei* [Sch06, Chapter 9].

Each skeletal muscle fiber is activated (made to contract) by one single motoneuron; however, a motoneuron can control a varying number of muscle fibers. The union of a motoneuron and the associated muscle fibers is called a *motor unit*

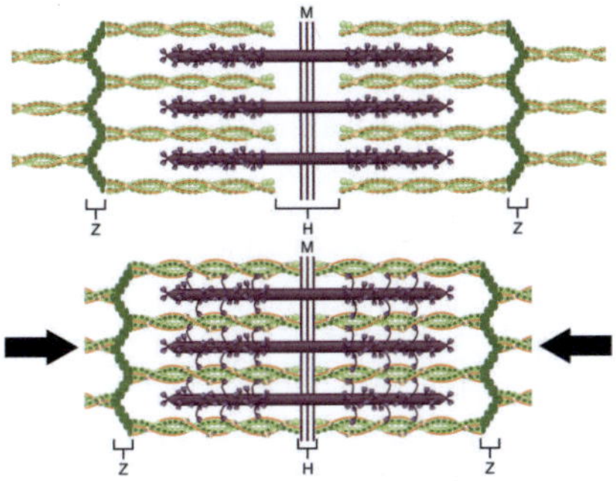

Figure 2.3 – Microstructure of muscle filaments (from [Col], CC-BY-3.0 license). The violet *Myosin* filaments slide along the green *Actin* filaments.

(MU). In case of the extraocular muscles, which require a very fine-grained control, one motoneuron controls 10 to 15 muscle fibers, whereas for the leg muscles, up to 5000 muscle fibers are controlled by one motoneuron [MP04]. Similarly, the number of motor units per muscle varies, numbers between 100 and 1000 are reported [BS80].

Since a motor unit is controlled by one single motoneuron, the associated muscle fibers are always activated in unison. When this happens, this motor unit is said to be *recruited.* In this case an action potential is generated. It propagates along the axon of the motoneuron, which branches close to the muscle and is connected to its associated muscle fibers at the *neuromuscular junctions.* A neuromuscular junction is a gap of around 30nm into which chemical transmitter substances are released when the motoneuron "fires": As with neurons, these transmitter substances cause the opening of ion channels in the muscle, inducing a *muscular action potential* based on positively charged ions. The action potential travels along the muscle fibers, sustaining and reinforcing itself. The involved ion types include K+, Na+, and Ca2+, the latter is primarily responsible for muscle contraction [Hop06].

The Contraction Cycle The constituting parts of the myofibril are *myosin* and *actin* filaments, which form an interlacing pattern in the myofibril, as depicted in figure 2.3. This structure is called a *sarcomere.*

The myosin molecule exhibits a specific structure, whose key part is the *head,* which can link with the actin filament. During a contraction process, the myosin heads enter a cycle in which they connect to actin filaments, change their shape so that the sarcomere shortens, and then disconnect from the actin filament.

So the myosin filaments "slide" along the actin filaments, giving this sequence the name *Sliding Filament Model* [Hux00]. The necessary energy is provided by a chemical reaction of the myosin head and the Adenosine triphosphate (ATP) molecule, available from the blood stream.

The contraction cycle is initiated by a chemical reaction involving the Ca2+ ions which are set free due to an incoming action potential. For a perceivable muscle shortening, the cycle must be repeated a large number of times. This repeated muscle activation stems from the sequence of incoming action potentials, so an increased activation frequency of the motoneuron directly causes the connected muscle fibers to generate more power. Furthermore, muscle power is regulated by the number of recruited motor units: these two principles account for the fine control of muscular force generation [MBSY73].

2.1.2 The Myoelectric Signal

Capturing Bioelectric Signals The human body produces a wide variety of electrical activity, ranging from strong potentials like the electrocardiac signal coming from heart activity to the small currents of neurons in the brain. These signals can be captured with *electrodes.*

Currents and potentials in the human body are produced by *ion* flows. Yet, technical systems require *electron* currents for processing. In the biophysiological context, electrodes are systems whose purpose is the conversion of ion flows into electron currents. They may take different forms: in particular, for medical uses of electromyography *indwelling* or *needle* electrodes are distinguished from *surface* electrodes [FC86]. Further electrode types are possible, ranging from *intracortical* electrodes which capture brain activity directly from the cortex [KWV00] to contactless *capacitative* electrodes [KHM05]. Application of needle electrodes requires penetrating the human skin, which introduces discomfort and infection risk. Furthermore, when measuring the EMG signal, typical needle electrodes impede the normal contraction of the muscle. Therefore, indwelling electrodes are mostly used in clinical contexts, e.g. to detect pathological changes in the neural innervation of the muscle [NWL08]. The remainder of this study only considers surface electrodes.

Typical surface electrodes used for signals like electromyography or electroencephalography are silver-silver chloride (Ag-AgCl) electrodes. This means that a solid body consisting of silver is covered with the corresponding salt (i.e. silver chloride). When such an electrode touches a liquid, the metal phase and the liquid phase enter into a chemical reaction, which makes the metal body release ions into the liquid. Since the chemical potentials of the two phases are different, an electric potential difference emerges between them. The simplest description of this process is the *Helmholtz Double Layer* model, which treats the phase boundary as an electrical capacitor [Kra07, Chapter 11]. At this phase boundary, the conversion of ion current and electrical current takes place.

Electrodes can be constructed to work on the bare skin, however this implies a very high transfer resistance between electrode and skin, making high-quality data capturing difficult. For this reason, typical electrodes, including the ones used for the experiments reported in this thesis, require application of a *conductive gel* between electrode and skin, which contains a solution of natrium chloride (NaCl) salt. The overall properties of the electrode are thus determined by the chemical properties of the metal (i.e. silver) and halogen (i.e. chloride) which constitute the electrode, and the conductive gel.

Since electrodes measure a potential difference, any measurement requires at least two electrodes. There are two main ways of deriving any such signal [FC86]: *Unipolar derivation* means that one electrode is placed at a position where a signal is to be measured, and the other electrode is placed at a neutral point (for Electromyography, this might be above a bone, i.e. at a place without muscular activity). *Bipolar derivation* means that two electrodes are placed on active surface (above a muscle), close to each other. The advantage of this approach is that certain artifacts (in particular, disturbance from electrical activity in the surroundings) cause identical activity at both electrodes: since the difference of the two potentials is measured, such artifacts are automatically suppressed.

In both forms of derivation, the signal from the two electrodes is fed into a differential amplifier, A/D converted and can then be further processed by a digital computer. Of course, in many practical scenarios a larger number of channels and thus electrodes is required.

Electromyography: Measurement of Muscular Activity Measuring muscle activity is a classical application of electrode technology. Ag/AgCl electrodes are attached above a muscle in either unipolar or bipolar configuration, in the latter case, it is imperative to place the electrodes along the direction of the muscle fibers, so that action potentials within muscle fibers are correctly captured.

As described in section 2.1, during contraction each muscle fiber exhibits its own action potential. However, since all fibers of a motor unit are activated simultaneously, the smallest unit of electrical muscle activity which can *in principle* be observed by surface electromyography is the summation of the action potentials of the fibers of the activated motor unit, a so-called *Motor Unit Action Potential* (MUAP) [dL79]. Since muscle contraction requires a sequence of action potentials, one obtains a sequence of MUAPs, a so-called *Motor Unit Action Potential Train* (MUAPT).

A typical EMG signal consists of the superposition of a multitude of MUAPTs, originating from different sources within a muscle and even from different muscles, particularly in regions where many overlapping muscles are present (e.g. the face). Therefore the observed EMG signal attains properties of a stochastic process [FC86], making its interpretation a challenging task. Detecting and separating MUAPTs is a primary concern in healthcare- and physiology-related applications of electromyography [LL82, LXL82, NWL08, dLAW$^+$06].

As described in chapter 4, our method of interpreting EMG signals uses a different principle. It is not the goal to break down the EMG signal into its constituing MUAPs, which for facial EMG signals is a formidable task [dLAW$^+$06]. Instead, the approach is based on pattern matching: the facial EMG signals are processed by a classifier in order to obtain the underlying speech, without making the attempt to fully trace back the sources of the observed activity.

2.1.3 Artifacts and Challenges

In bioelectrical signals, *artifacts* are interfering voltages which distort the measured signal [Kra07, Chapter 11]. They may be caused by a variety of factors related to the measured subject (biological artifacts) and the technology (technical artifacts).

Technical artifacts are caused for example by amplification noise, bad electrical contact points (e.g. between electrodes and amplifier), and interference from external power sources, which is usually observed as a strong 50 Hz or 60 Hz frequency component in the signal. Causes for biological artifacts in the EMG signal include movements of the user and sweating, ECG interspersion (i.e. heart activity) is sometimes also observed.

Defining the term "artifact" liberally, deteriorated signal quality is furthermore caused by the peculiarities of the intended application. In the face, capturing EMG by means of surface electrodes necessarily implies that each electrode captures signals from several muscles. If information about a particular muscle is desired, this *cross-talk* may be considered an artifact as well. Additionally, signal distortions in EMG-based speech recognition are caused by facial movements which are not related to speaking, like swallowing, chewing, smiling, etc.

All these artifacts are detrimental to optimal signal quality and recognizer performance. Application-related artifacts can be minimized by careful setup and recording procedures, for example, our subjects were asked to avoid extraneous facial movements. Technical artifacts are reduced by using high-quality components, and by assuring optimal recording conditions, for example locations with low electrical interference. Biological artifacts are similarly avoided e.g. by using air-conditioned rooms for recording. Still, artifacts necessarily occur, and artifact detection and reduction is one particular application of the new EMG array technology described in chapter 7.

2.1.4 Applications of Electromyography

Electromyography is an established technology with a multitude of applications. A classical one is medical diagnosis and treatment: Muscle contraction behavior can be checked using electromyography in order to discover muscle pathologies. This extends to the study of the neuromuscular pathways, i.e. the connections between a patient's brain and body, and allows diagnosis of a variety of diseases of the brain and nervous system, including Parkinson's disease, cerebral palsy, and stroke [dLAW+06]. For these applications, one frequently uses a *decomposition* of the EMG signal into its constituent MUAPTs [LL82, LXL82, NWL08, HZ07], also see the further background notes in chapter 7. A whole tome about the topic of EMG-based analysis of neuromuscular disorders is [PS12].

The planning and execution of movements has also been studied by electromyography (clearly, if any form of extensive movement is involved, EMG is necessarily captured by surface electrodes). Such investigations deal with a variety of settings: from competitive sports to everyday life, from healthy people to disabled persons, etc. [CC93] offers an extensive review.

EMG is furthermore applied in rehabilitation, ergonomics, and biofeedback, just to name some more examples from medicine and physiology. An extensive treatment is found in [MP04, Chapters 12 - 17].

In this study, we are particularly interested in machine-learning related uses of EMG. Since EMG is a biosignal which can be generated even by a large group of physically handicapped patients, assistive technologies easily come to mind. We mention in particular the control of limb prostheses with electromyography [CvdS09, SG82, EHP01], [MP04, Chapter 18]: Here the goal is to control, as naturally as possible, an artificial arm or leg. Unfortunately, as explained in [CvdS09], fully intuitively control of prostheses with a large number of degrees of freedom has not yet been realized. Yet, investigations on this topic are progressing speedily, driven by recent advances both in EMG recording hardware and real-time classification techniques.

The myoelectric signal is also used as the basis of human-computer interfaces (HCI), and the research conducted for this thesis falls into this category. From a pattern recognition standpoint, current applications in assistive technologies for disabled patients are frequently limited to relatively simple setups, where a few distinct commands e.g. for controlling a computer mouse are distinguished [MLM04, BSA00]. In this study we present an HCI based on speech recognition by facial electromyography: This is clearly a far more complex machine learning task, since a high number of different activity patterns have to be recognized in order to discern speech.

2.2 Speech Production and Perception

Physically, sound can be described as a superposition of *pressure waves* moving through a medium. The term "pressure wave" means that the wave is formed by compressions and rarefactions of the molecules of the medium. Since these compressions occur in the direction of the propagation of the pressure wave, sound waves are *longitudinal waves.* Like any physical wave, the sound pressure wave can be described by a sine function, where by definition locations of maximal compression correspond to maxima of the sine, and locations of maximal rarefaction correspond to minima of the sine (see figure 2.4).

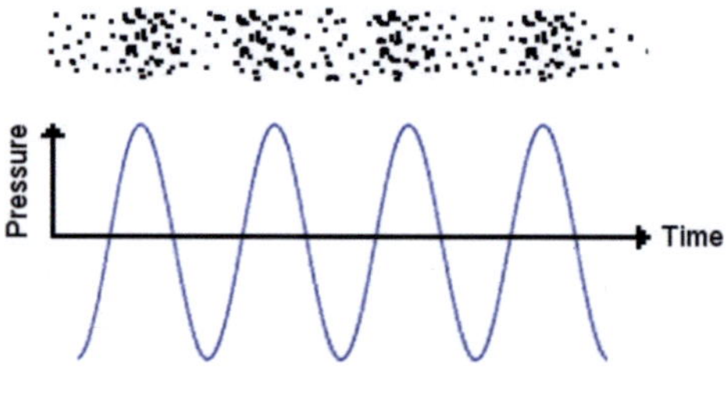

Figure 2.4 – Sound as a Pressure Wave. The sound wave may be described by a part of a sine function, where by definition locations of maximal compression correspond to maxima of the sine, and locations of maximal rarefaction correspond to minima of the sine.

This exposition only considers sound waves propagating through air, since this is the scenario in which spoken communication occurs. In this case, the propagatation speed is approximately $331.5 + 0.6T\frac{m}{s}$, where T is the temperature, measured in degrees Celsius [HAH01, Chapter 2.1]. It should be noted that the air molecules participating in the sound wave are not transported along with the wave, they just oscillate around their resting position.

The amplitude of the sound wave, as shown in figure 2.4, corresponds to the amount of energy needed for displacing the molecules. This amount of energy is related to the perceived loudness of the sound wave, however the relationship is quite complex [Ols72]. While the human ear can normally perceive sounds of up to 20kHz (substantially decreasing with age), the bandwidth necessary for understanding human speech has a far lower upper limit; a maximal frequency of 8kHz is considered sufficient. This gives rise to a standard speech sampling rate of 16 kHz. It can be shown that the most speech signal energy is found at frequencies even below 8kHz, as an example, consider figure 2.9, which shows *spectrograms* of two speech signals (once whispered, once normally spoken). Particularly in the case of normal speech, it is obvious that most signal energy is found in the lower half of the spectrogram, i.e. below 4kHz. For more details on speech sounds, please refer to section 2.2.2.

In section 2.2.1 it is described how speech sounds are produced. Otherwise, we are interested in the high-level properties of human speech: Section 2.2.2 explains how the large variation in human speech sounds is possible. Section 2.2.3 describes the *speaking modes* which are used in this thesis: audible, whispered, and silent speech. Finally, in section 2.2.4 we report on speech perception.

2.2.1 Anatomy of the Speech Production System

Human speech is produced by the articulatory apparatus, which is shown in figure 2.5. The air pressure waves which form human speech are created in the lungs, they then pass the *larynx* and the *vocal tract*, where they undergo complex modifications which account for the variety of speech sounds, and finally emanate from the mouth and the nostrils of the speaker.

In the lungs, air pressure is built up. The first organ which modulates the airstream and influences the produced speech sounds are the *vocal chords*, located in the *larynx*. The *glottis* is defined as the combination of vocal chords and the space enclosed by them.

If the vocal chords are held tense, so that the airflow sets them into vibration, a *voiced* sound is created. The main characteristic of this sound is the *fundamental frequency*, which is the frequency at which the vocal chords vibrate; it ranges from 60 Hz for a large man to as high as 300 Hz for a small woman or a child [HAH01]. The fundamental frequency is determined by the length and the tautness of the vocal chords, so it can be varied in a certain range. This gives rise to *intonation*, which plays an important role in speech perception. The waveform

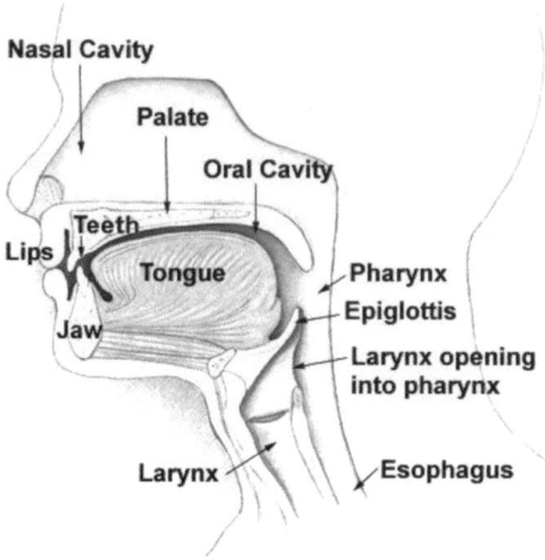

Figure 2.5 – Schematic diagram of the human articulatory apparatus (adapted from [USNIoHa], public domain)

generated by the vocal chords exhibits further frequencies, namely the *harmonics* (integer multiples) of the fundamental frequency.

If the vocal chords are held slack, so that they do not vibrate, an *unvoiced* sound is generated. This sound may be described as an audible turbulence without discernible fundamental frequency: instead, a broad spectrum of high-frequency components is observed, closely resembling *white noise*[1].

After leaving the glottis, the airstream passes through the *vocal tract*, consisting of the oral and nasal cavity, and the articulators therein (tongue, lips, etc.). While the glottis creates the speech excitation, and thus the distinction between voiced and unvoiced sounds, the vocal tract is where the majority of speech sound modulation takes place. Section 2.2.2 reports on the mechanisms the vocal tract uses for this purpose.

The process of speech sound generation is frequently described with the *source-filter model*, see figure 2.6. It consists of a sound source (the glottis), creating either voiced or unvoiced excitation, and a filter (the vocal tract), modifying the excitation signal. Mathematically, a *filter* boosts or attenuates certain frequencies of the input signal, so that in frequency domain, it can be described as a simple multiplication [SH90]. This is expressed by formula (2.1) describing the

[1]The turbulent noise emanating from the glottis as the basic excitation of unvoiced sounds should not be confused with the audible turbulence when a (voiced or unvoiced) *fricative* sound is pronounced: In the former case, the turbulence is created by the glottis, in the latter case, the turbulence is due to constrictions in the vocal tract.

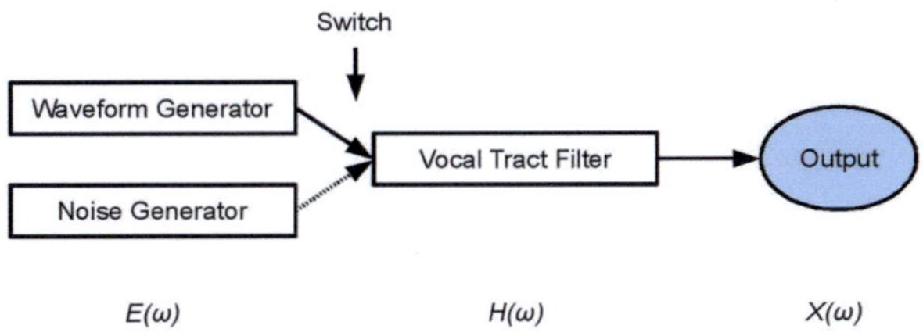

Figure 2.6 – The source-filter model of speech production

the source-filter model: In frequency domain, the speech signal $X(\omega)$, i.e. the output of the vocal tract, is computed from the excitation $E(\omega)$ and the vocal tract frequency response $H(\omega)$ with the formula

$$X(\omega) = E(\omega) \cdot H(\omega). \tag{2.1}$$

Describing the vocal tract as a mathematical filter is quite accurate for vowels, i.e. sounds which are produced without a constriction in the vocal tract, however the airstream modifications for consonant generation cannot be described by filters alone. Nonetheless, the source-filter model is widely used since it is simple and effective.

2.2.2 Phonetics and Phonology

Speech sounds (or *phones*) are generated from the voiced or unvoiced excitation by the interplay of the articulators. Different sounds result from different configurations of the articulators, modifying the airstream in a variety of ways. Phones can roughly be divided into two basic classes [HAH01]:

- *Vowels* are articulated without major constrictions in the vocal tract. In this case, the vocal tract acts as a filter: the most strongly emphasized frequencies are called *formants*, they unambiguously characterize a vowel sound. Vowels are always voiced. It is possible to articulate continuous transitions between vowels, giving rise to *diphthongs* and even *triphthongs*.
- Articulation of *Consonants* is characterized by a constriction in the vocal tract. This constriction may take several forms, giving rise to a set of very different speech sounds, as described below. Consonants can be voiced or unvoiced.

Since a vowel is pronounced with a vocal tract free of (major) obstructions, the main factor in determining its sound is the position of the tongue. Furthermore,

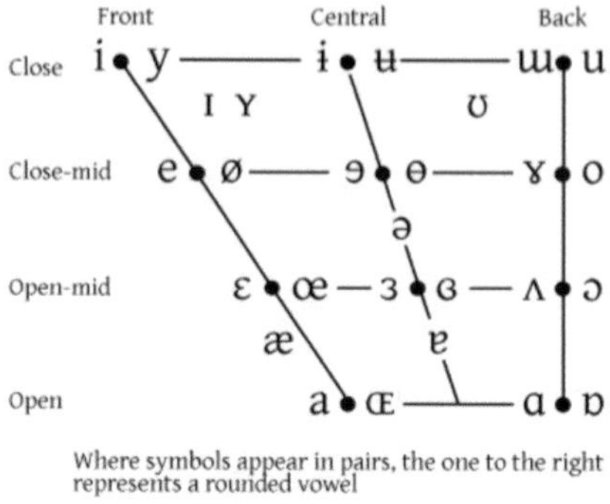

Figure 2.7 – IPA vowel quadrangle [Int99]

lip rounding changes vowel characteristics, and in the case of *nasal vowels*, which exist in languages like French and Portuguese, air emerges through both mouth and nose. Thus, we have four main parameters describing vowel articulation: Vertical and horizontal tongue position, lip rounding, and nasalization.

Vowels are frequently described by the *vowel quadrangle*, which is shown in figure 2.7. The symbols are part of the *International Phonetic Alphabet* [Int99], which has been developed in order to provide a unified notation for all possible speech sounds, of all possible languages. In the vowel quadrangle, three of the four main properties are shown: the *closeness* or *height* (vertical position of the tongue), the *backness* (horizontal position of the tongue), and the *rounding* of the lips.

Closeness and backness are charted on the vertical and horizontal axis, respectively, and it becomes clear that these are actually *continuous* variables; yet in order to be able to write vowels as discrete symbols, the standard IPA alphabet only distinguishes seven vowel heights and five degrees of vowel backness. The third dimension, given by pairs of symbols, signifies the roundedness of the lips. Nasalization is not shown in the basic IPA vowel chart, in writing it is indicated with a tilde symbol over the vowel.

For consonants, a classification scheme based on the vocal tract obstruction is used. The main factors in describing a consonant are the *manner* of articulation, the *position* of articulation, and *voicing*. Possible manners of articulation are as follows:

- *Fricatives* are produced by forcing the airflow through a narrow gap between two articulators put close to each other, for example, pronouncing the phone [f] involves the upper lip and the lower teeth

CONSONANTS (PULMONIC)

	Bilabial	Labiodental	Dental	Alveolar	Postalveolar	Retroflex	Palatal	Velar	Uvular	Pharyngeal	Glottal
Plosive	p b			t d		ʈ ɖ	c ɟ	k ɡ	q ɢ		ʔ
Nasal	m	ɱ		n		ɳ	ɲ	ŋ	ɴ		
Trill	ʙ			r					ʀ		
Tap or Flap				ɾ		ɽ					
Fricative	ɸ β	f v	θ ð	s z	ʃ ʒ	ʂ ʐ	ç ʝ	x ɣ	χ ʁ	ħ ʕ	h ɦ
Lateral fricative				ɬ ɮ							
Approximant		ʋ		ɹ		ɻ	j	ɰ			
Lateral approximant				l		ɭ	ʎ	ʟ			

Where symbols appear in pairs, the one to the right represents a voiced consonant. Shaded areas denote articulations judged impossible.

Figure 2.8 – IPA chart for consonants [Int99]

- *Plosives* are produced by shortly stopping the airflow altogether, as for the phone [p], where the lips close off the airstream
- *Approximants* are produced when two articulators are placed close to each other, but not close enough to create turbulence as in the fricative case. Examples (in English language) include the phones [l] and [r], as well as *semivowels* like [y] as in "yes"
- *Lateral* sounds, e.g. [l], are produced by blocking the central oral cavity with the tongue, so that air emerges along the *side* of the tongue.
- *Nasals* like [m] and [n] are produced by closing off the oral cavity, letting air emerge through the nose only. They must be distinguished from nasal vowels, where air emerges from mouth *and* nose simultaneously
- *Flaps* occur when an active articulator shortly hits a passive one. In contrast to a plosive sound, no air pressure is built up behind the place where the articulators connect.
- *Trill* sounds, like the Spanish trilled [ṙ], are airstream-caused periodic vibrations of an articulator.

The articulation position is the point of main constriction, ranging from *bilabial* (for sounds which are produced with the lips, like [b] and [p]) to *glottal* (main constriction at the glottis, like [h]). Voicedness is the third distinctive feature of consonants, many of which exist in voiced/unvoiced pairs, like e.g. [t] and [d]. The set of consonants is represented in the consonant table from the IPA chart (figure 2.8), with manner of articulation on the vertical axis, position of articulation on the horizontal axis, and paired symbols representing a pair of voiced and unvoiced consonants.

One observes from figures 2.5 and 2.8 that most articulation positions can be directly associated with articulators, for example, there are bilabial consonants which are formed with the lips, dental and alveolar consonants which are formed with the teeth resp. the tooth ridge (alveolar ridge), etc. The tongue frequently plays an important role as well. The exception to this rule are *retroflex* consonants, which are characterized not by a concrete position of articulation, but instead by being articulated with a curled tongue; they are rare in European languages.

Properties like place or manner of articulation, or the tongue position from the vowel quadrangle, are called *phonetic* or *articulatory features* [Kir99]. In this study we prefer the term *phonetic features* (PFs) since these properties are not directly derived from the movement of the articulators, but rather from the study of phonetics. In this thesis, phonetic features play a key role in the modeling for the EMG-based spech recognizer, see chapter 5.

Of course, no existing language uses *all* possible phones, and even if a subset of phones exist in a given language, not all existing phone contrasts cause differences in the meaning of words. Therefore, phonetics distinguishes phones from *phonemes*: while phones differ in their acoustic realization, phonemes convey meaning differences. If a pair of words which just differ by one phone exists, these phones are realizations of different phonemes: for example, in the English language, [b] and [p] are different phonemes since the words "bill" and "pill" are different. A word pair like "bill"/"pill" which only differs by one phone is called *minimal pair.*

A phoneme may be realized by different phones, so-called *allophones*: For example, in the English language the phoneme /l/[2] has at least two allophones, namely the voiced lateral-alveolar approximant [l] as in "lip" and the velarized "dark l" [ɫ] as in "pill". Finally, we note that phonemes are strongly language-dependent, whereas phones may to a certain extent be shared between languages (this is a key requirement for building multilingual speech recognition systems [Sch00]).

2.2.3 *Speaking Modes*: Whispered and Silent Speech

So far, we have described normally spoken, or *audible* speech. This thesis aims at enabling speech communication with the special purpose of communicating

[2]Phonemes are commonly written between slashes, like /l/, phones are written in square brackets, like [l].

covertly, without disturbing bystanders or compromising confidentiality. For this purpose, we investigate both *whispered* and *silent* speech, we particularly focus on the difference between these *speaking modes* in chapter 6.

Whispered speech is a speaking mode which consists entirely of unvoiced speech, so for all voiced phones, the excitation signal created by the vibrating vocal chords is replaced by a voiceless turbulence. Since whispered speech is intended for communicating privately, it is typically pronounced more quietly than normal speech, so that it is only audible in a very close vicinity. Yet, unperturbed whispered speech evidently carries all information necessary for understanding its content; it is also notable that minimal pairs which only differ in the voicing of a single phone may still be distinguished in whispered speech [Dan80].

The phonetic properties of whispered speech and audible speech diverge to a certain extent, caused by the different excitation signal, but also by the changed configuration of the vocal tract which is necessary to prevent the vocal chords from vibrating. Typical differences are (taken from [ITI05], see also the references therein):

- The signal energy is lower in whispered speech than in audible speech, particularly for lower frequencies (which in audible speech carry the main energy of the signal)
- The *formant frequencies* of the vowels shift upwards, and likewise, the formant boundaries between vowels change
- Voiceless consonants are least affected by switching from audible to whispered speech, and vowels are most affected: This causes the notable result that in whispered speech, vowels do no more bear the main energy of the signal, as they do in normal, audible speech.

Further differences have been observed, for example, the duration of certain phones or syllables is increased in whispered speech [Sch72]. For a listing of more studies regarding the phonological difference between whispered and normal speech, we refer to the comprehensive background information in [Osf11].

Whispered speech has mostly been studied acoustically. Yet, research based on other methods exists: H. Yoshioka collected electropalatographical recordings of whispered speech [Yos08], measuring tongue contact patterns for the two phones /s/ and /z/ in whispered speech. Higashikawa et al. performed kinematic measurements of the jaw opening [HGMM03]. Whispered speech has also been considered for acoustic speech recognition, here it is observed that recognition across speaking modes requires several special adaptation steps [ITI05, JSW04, Jou08]. However to our knowledge, there exist no studies which deal with the articulation of whispered speech at the muscle level, or with the manifestation of the whispered speaking mode in the facial EMG signal.

We define ***Silent Speech*** as follows: The speaker is told to move the articulators as normally as possible, while suppressing the pulmonary airstream, so that no sound is heard.

During our recordings, we made two major observations. First, it is often difficult to produce *totally* silent speech. This applies in particular to plosive consonants and fricatives, where the process of articulation fundamentally depends on an airstream. Some of our subjects reacted to this problem by producing these sounds in a very quiet whisper, which our recording supervisors corrected as soon as these whispers became understandable. However, as long as no complete words could be discerned in silent speech recordings, very quiet articulation sounds were not rejected. Those subjects who managed to articulate silent speech without actually producing any sound at all frequently reported that they felt that their articulation of certain sounds, particularly plosives, changed drastically compared to audible speech.

The second observation relates to Silent Speech consistency. Inconsistencies are expected for two reasons: first, our subjects did not have any experience in speaking silently, and second, auditory feedback, which plays a major role in normal articulation (see section 6.1 for more details), fails for silent speech. A particular inconsistency which was corrected by the recording supervisors as soon as it was observed is loss of articulatory movements: When an (inexperienced) subject spoke silently over several minutes, sometimes his or her articulatory movements became less and less pronounced, disappearing almost completely over time if the supervisor did not intervene. Clearly, this is a problem when silent speech is produced by inexperienced persons. We ran some initial experiments on giving *feedback* to our subjects during the recording of silent speech, in order to devise an automatic method to avoid such issues. However none of the investigated methods was robust enough to be made the basis of a large-scale recording [HJWS11].

As a final remark on silent speech, we report that several studies regarding speech production by hearing-impaired persons exist (for example, [OM82]). These studies clearly show that when a person does not hear his or her own voice, the properties of the produced speech change. Yet, we assume that these results do not fully carry over to silently *produced* speech, since not only auditory feedback is missing, but the process of articulation itself is affected.

Silent speech can (unfortunately) not be studied acoustically (in chapter 6, we investigate the articulation differences between silent and audible speech at EMG signal level). However, it is instructive to visualize whispered and audible

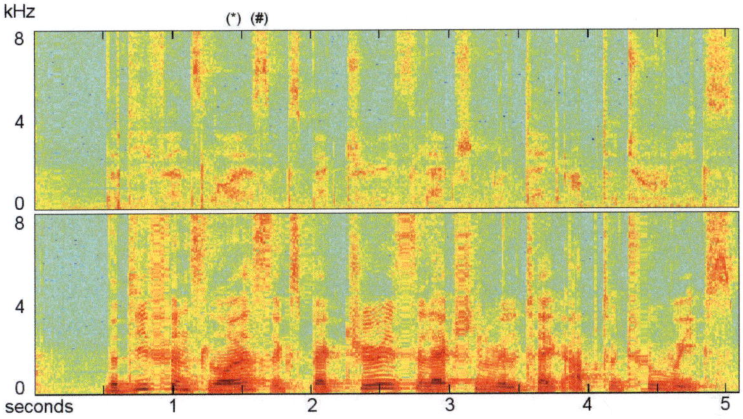

Figure 2.9 – Exemplary spectra of the sentence "The defense lawyers expect jury selection will take up to two weeks", whispered (above) and normally spoken (below). The spectrograms are aligned for comparability. The mark (*) indicates a typical vowel, the mark (#) indicate a fricative.

speech. A classical speech representation is the *spectrogram*, where the speech signal is divided into frames, and the frequency components of the frames are plotted over time. Figure 2.9 shows logarithmized spectrograms of the sentence "The defense lawyers expect jury selection will take up to two weeks", once whispered (above), once normally spoken (below).

Two typical speech sounds which are easily visually distinguished are highlighted: The mark (*) indicates a vowel, in the lower spectrogram, where normal speech is displayed, the fundamental frequency and its multiples are recognizable as "ripples". The formant coutours can be seen as maxima over the spectrum; they are also visible in the whispered speech spectrogram, however a fundamental frequency contour does not exist. At position (#), a typical voiced fricative (the [z] from the word "lawyers") is seen. Again, in the audible speech spectrogram the fundamental frequency multiples are seen as ripples, and for both audible and whispered speech, a high-frequency noise indicates the presence of a fricative.

2.2.4 Speech Perception

For the purpose of this thesis, the productional aspect of speech plays a more important role than the perceptional aspect. Still, speech perception is a central aspect when dealing with speech recognition, and within the context of this thesis, it is relevant to the question of articulatory control, as detailed in section 6.1. Therefore this part contains a short summary of the properties and functionality of the human ear.

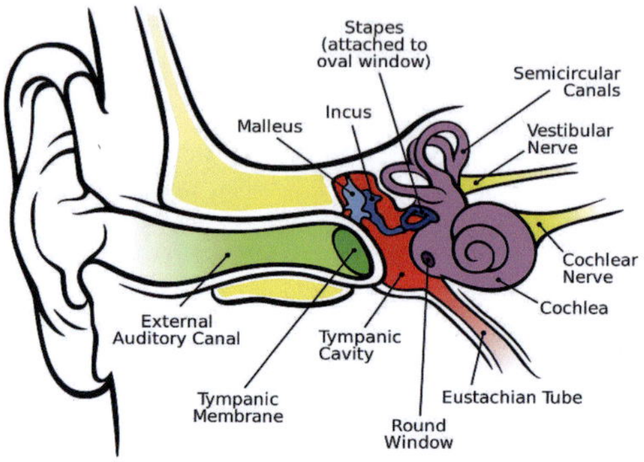

Figure 2.10 – The ear (from [Wik13a], CC-BY-2.5 license)

Figure 2.10 shows the anatomy of the human ear, which is divided into three parts—the *outer ear*, which collects incoming sounds, the *middle ear*, which amplifies the sound wave, and the *inner ear*, where sounds are converted into nerve impulses, thus being usable as an input to the brain.

The outer ear collects sound waves, for which its cup-like form is optimized. The collected waves pass through the *auditory canal* to the middle ear, which is delimited by the *tympanic membrane*. The middle ear has a twofold function: It acts as an amplifier, and the sound wave is converted from an air wave into a fluid wave, i.e. a wave in a liquid medium. This conversion and amplification is performed by the three *auditory ossicles*, which are small bones located within the middle ear.

The auditory ossicles transfer the speech waveform to the inner ear, whose main component is the spiral-shaped *cochlea*. Here, the *hair cells* are found, which are excited by the incoming fluid sound waves. Different hair cells are excited by different frequencies (this stems from variations in their diameter and stiffness), so that the inner ear essentially performs a frequency decomposition of the sound signal. The hair cells are directly connected to the *cochlear* (or *auditory*) nerve, which links the ear to the brain.

Thus, humans (and many animals) perform hearing by mechanically generating a frequency decomposition of incoming sounds. This observation gave rise to several common signal preprocessing algorithms in acoustic speech recognition, which are often based on the Fourier transform, see section 2.3.1.

2.3 Introduction to Automatic Speech Recognition

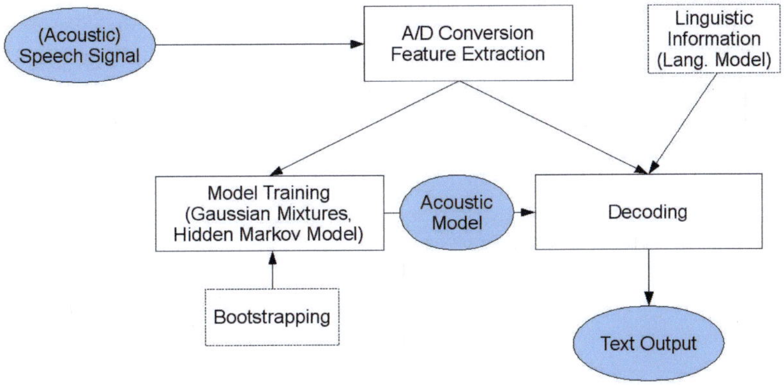

Figure 2.11 – Components of a traditional speech recognizer. The processing chain starts with speech input (upper left), which is used to train the *acoustic model.* When the acoustic model has been created, speech can be decoded, yielding text output (lower right).

A significant part of this study, as well as of prior studies (e.g. [Jou08]), deals with adapting the standard speech recognition chain towards the properties of the EMG signal and the EMG representation of the process of speaking (audibly or silently). Therefore this chapter contains a walkthrough of standard speech recognition, with the purpose of serving as a reference point in later chapters. Also note that an acoustic speech recognizer is used for a process we call *label bootstrapping*: The models of the EMG-based speech recognizer are initialized from scratch, with the help of time-alignments (or labels) created from the acoustic signal; see section 4.1.1 for more information.

Figure 2.11 presents the components of a classical speech recognizer. The speech signals which serve as input are recorded with any type of microphone and A/D converted (digitalized) for further processing. Usually sampling is performed at 16kHz. We always use read speech as input for training and testing, which is divided into *utterances*, i.e. short recordings of speech in the approximate length of one sentence. We assume throughout this thesis that the textual content of the utterances, the *transcription*, is known and accurate, with the only exception of *unsupervised* session adaptation, see section 8.2.3.

After digitalization, *features* are extracted, which represent the speech signal in a manner suitable for classification. The next step is the *training* of the recognizer: Here a set of training data is processed to generate *models* of acoustic units (for example, phones). The collection of all model information extracted from the training data is called the *acoustic model*; consequently, in this thesis we introduce the term ***myoelectric model*** to describe all information in the trained recognizer which stems from the EMG input signal. Finally, when the acoustic model has been created, *decoding* can be performed on (unknown) speech input, yielding a *hypothesis* of the textual content of the spoken utterance. During this process, the *language model* yields a priori information about the likelihood of certain sequences of words, irrespective of the acoustic signal. Finally, the *(pronunciation) dictionary* (not shown in figure 2.11) contains pronunciations for all words occurring during training and decoding. Thus it has the important role of linking words and their pronunciations. While in contemporary large-vocabulary speech recognition dictionary creation can be a daunting task, for this thesis a fixed dictionary is used, which is described in section 4.

2.3.1 Acoustic Feature Extraction

The raw speech waveform is not directly useful for speech recognition and processing: it contains too much redundant and superfluous information, and the relevant information is not readily available. In particular, a *single* amplitude value *by itself* contains almost no usable information.

Feature extraction aims at emphasizing signal properties relevant for speech sound classification, while reducing redundant information. Furthermore, the speech signal is an (albeit highly-sampled) *continuous* signal, from which a *discrete* sequence of phones is to be recognized. Therefore, one step of acoustic feature extraction is *framing* or *windowing*: The signal is divided into short time segments, and from each of these segments a single feature vector is extracted, thus discretizing the time dimension of the speech signal on a coarse scale. The output of feature extraction is a matrix of dimensionality $N \times D$, where D is the dimension of each feature vector, and N is the number of time frames. We use the convention that time runs from top to bottom, so each *row* of the matrix is a D-dimensional feature vector.

Speech feature extraction has been researched for many decades; here we present *Mel Frequency Cepstral Coefficients* (MFCC) as a contemporary standard. MFCC feature extraction consists of the following steps:

- The speech signal is divided into *frames* with a frame width of 16ms and a frame shift of 10ms. This frame shift is a long-established standard, it reflects the properties of phones: A phone is assumed to last at least 30ms, which then amounts to three frames. These are allowed to be acoustically different (consider, for example, a plosive sound, which consists of a short silence followed by a burst and an aspiration). A longer frameshift would preclude subdividing a phone into parts, a shorter frameshift brings no further improvement, but increases the computation time.
- Each frame is multiplied with a Hamming window [Ham89] to reduce distortion in the following step:
- The frame-wise spectrum is computed by the Discrete Fourier Transform.

Thus we have obtained a discrete representation of the speech signal in the frequency domain. The idea of using a frequency representation is motivated by the properties of the human ear, see section 2.2.4.

- A *filterbank* is used for dimensionality reduction. This means that weighted averages over adjacent frequency components are computed, such that the total number of coefficients in the feature vector is reduced. The number and shape of the filters is determined by perceptional considerations: The human ear distinguishes lower frequencies at a much finer scale than higher frequencies. This gives rise to the Mel scale [SVN37], which ranks *perceived* pitch versus *actual* frequency. The conversion is approximately logarithmic, i.e. at high frequencies, the perceived pitch rises much more slowly than the actual frequency. Therefore, the Mel filterbank consists of a set of triangular filters, where filters at lower frequencies are much denser and more narrow than filters at high frequencies. Typical numbers of Mel filters range around 30. For a more general treatment of dimensionality reduction see section 2.4.
- The logarithm of the frame-wise Mel spectra is taken, then each frame is processed with the discrete cosine transform (alternatively, the Discrete Fourier Transform can be used), transforming the features into *Cepstral Domain*. This step amounts to a *deconvolution* of the excitation source and the vocal tract filter (compare the source-filter model of speech production described in section 2.2.1).
- Of the resulting representation, the first 13 coefficients per frame are kept, again reducing the signal dimensionality. Optionally, context information can be modeled by stacking adjacent feature frames. The context width can be varied e.g. between 1 and 10. If higher context widths are used, Lin-

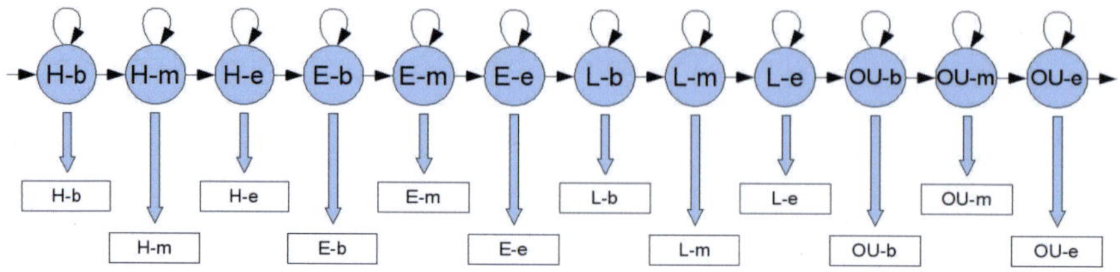

Figure 2.12 – Three-state context-independent phone HMM for the word "Hello". The upper row of circles indicates the possible sequence of states, the lower row of rectangles shows the emission probabilities.

ear Discriminant Analysis (LDA) (see section 2.4) should be applied after stacking in order to perform dimensionality reduction.

MFCCs are quickly computed and are known to give good recognition results. It is clear that they are based on a frequency decomposition of the speech signal, but go well beyond a simple application of the Fourier transform, since they take speech perception into account.

2.3.2 Unit Modeling and Sequence Modeling

We define a *model* as a stochastic representation of certain properties of the (speech) input signal. Here we deal with the *acoustic model*, which represents the acoustic properties of speech, i.e. the acoustic realization of phones and phonemes, and the possible sequences of phones which make up the words of the *vocabulary*. As we mentioned above, the language model, which assigns probabilities to sequences of words, and the dictionary, which maps words to phone sequences, are additional knowledge sources, see section 2.3.6.

The model structure is a key design decision when building a speech recognizer. Its importance stems from the requirement that one wishes to recognize a potentially unlimited set of words, even if these words do not appear in the training data set. Therefore, models of words must be composed from smaller units, for example from syllable models or phone models. The latter is the standard in speech recognition and is described in this section. Furthermore, the model structure has an impact on the extent of data sharing between word models, and consequently on the required amount of training data, it influences the computational efficiency of the algorithm, the ability to deal with coarticulation effects, accents, etc. Section 5 of this thesis presents a novel modeling approach for the EMG-based speech recognition system.

Formally the acoustic model consists of two parts, the *unit model* and the *sequence model*. We use the nonstandard term "unit model" to refer to the modeling of the acoustic properties of phones or phonetic features, which is done at the frame level. Sequence models determine the possible sequences of phones, up to word or utterance level.

In the simplest case, unit models represent phones or *subphones* (i.e. the beginning, middle, or end part of phones). They are usually based on Gaussian mixture models, see section 2.3.3; for now we only require that given any feature vector, a unit model is able to provide a probability that the feature vector matches the model[3].

Sequence modeling is normally performed with a *Hidden Markov Model* (HMM), which provides a framework for combining unit models into words and utterances. This is done by augmenting the unit models, which are ignorant of their context, with *transition probabilities* which model the probability with which a certain *sequence* of unit models occurs. For such kinds of models, the term *sequence models* has been coined.

In order to give an intuitive explanation of the HMM concept, consider figure 2.12. A model of the word "Hello" is shown, which according to the dictionary consists of the four phones [H], [E], [L], and [OU]. In general linguistic usage, such a single-utterance model is also called an "HMM", even though this is somewhat inaccurate since it is just a representation of a single utterance *within* the HMM.

The blue circles representing subphones are the *states* of the HMM. The further constituting parts are as follows:

- The *transition probabilities* are represented by the arrows connecting the HMM states. We did not label the arrows with probability values since practically all contemporary speech recognizers do not use different transition probabilities. Instead it is assumed that all transitions which are allowed are equally probable, and that the possibility of word sequences is determined by the language model. Transitions which are not indicated by arrows are impossible, for example, the HMM in figure 2.12 is *unable* to model the word "hole" ([H] [OU] [L]).
- The white rectangles assigned to the HMM states are the *unit models*. In the case of figure 2.12, there is a one-to-one correspondence between unit

[3]The mathematician might argue that Gaussian (mixture) models yield values of a probability density function, not true probabilities. This goes beyond the scope of this explanation and is of no concern anyway; yet, it might be more exact to say that a unit model must yield a scalar value describing how well a feature vector and the model match, this scalar value may or may not be a probability.

models and HMM state names, but we will see below that this is not always the case.

Thus, we see that the HMM links unit models, which describe feature vectors but do not "know" anything about the context in which they occur, and transition probabilities, which describe how phone or subphone units are composed into words, but rely on the unit models to actually match a feature vector sequence. Within the context of an HMM, the probability distributions yielded by the unit models are called *emission probabilities*[4].

Hidden Markov Modeling has evolved into a standard in acoustic speech recognition, having the great advantage that efficient algorithms for HMM-related problems are available. Out of these, we mention

- the *forward* algorithm, which allows to compute the probability of an utterance HMM given a sequence of feature vectors and thus constitutes a first step towards *decoding*, i.e. recognizing unknown speech.
- the *forward-backward* algorithm and its deterministic counterpart, the *Viterbi* algorithm, which are used to determine optimal assignments of HMM states and feature frames. Such as assignment is called a *path* through the HMM.

Due to space constraints, we do not present these algorithms in detail, instead we refer to standard literature: a textbook treatise of HMM theory and concepts, as well as a more formal definition, can be found in [HAH01, Chapter 8]. A good tutorial introduction into HMM-related algorithmics is [Rab89].

2.3.3 Gaussian Mixture Models

In this section we deal with the concrete design of unit models, namely with their standard realization as *Gaussian mixture models* (GMMs).

First consider a single Gaussian model in the $\mathbb{R}^D$, which is given by its *probability density function*

$$\mathcal{N}(x \mid \mu, \Sigma) = (2\pi)^{-\frac{D}{2}} |\Sigma|^{-\frac{1}{2}} \exp\left(-\frac{1}{2}(x-\mu)^T \Sigma^{-1} (x-\mu)\right). \tag{2.2}$$

The Gaussian distribution is completely determined by its two parameters, the *mean* μ and the *covariance matrix* Σ. One can intuitively visualize a Gaussian as a "bubble" in space, representing the location and the spreading of the data.

[4]This term stems from the concept of generative modeling, i.e. the HMM states *generate* observed feature vectors. Some background information is found in [Bis07, Chapter 1.5].

If a data set with an irregular distribution is to be modeled, a single Gaussian distribution is frequently not flexible enough.

GMMs are simple yet powerful models which solve this problem and are therefore often used, in particular, almost all contemporary acoustic speech recognizers are based on GMM unit modeling. It can be shown that GMMs are a reasonable approximation for *any* probability distribution [Bis07, Chapter 2.3.9]. We will also see that there are powerful and efficient algorithms for estimating their parameters, making GMMs a versatile modeling concept.

A GMM is a weighted sum of single Gaussians, thus its density function is given by

$$p_{\text{GMM}}(x \,|\, \mathbf{w}, \boldsymbol{\mu}, \boldsymbol{\Sigma}) = \sum_{k=1}^{K} w_k \mathcal{N}(x \,|\, \mu_k, \Sigma_k), \tag{2.3}$$

where $\boldsymbol{\mu} = \{\mu_1, \dots, \mu_K\}$ are the component means, $\boldsymbol{\Sigma} = \{\Sigma_1, \dots, \Sigma_K\}$ are the component covariance matrices, and $\mathbf{w} = \{w_1, \dots, w_K\}$ is the set of component weights, which are nonnegative and required to sum to one. The single Gaussian model is a special case of the Gaussian Mixture model, and it is clear that the GMM satisfies the key requirement which we stated for unit models, namely, that it is possible to compute the probability of a feature vector x given the model: This is done by evaluating $p_{\text{GMM}}(x)$.

When a recognizer based on GMMs is to be *trained*, one needs to estimate the model parameters, i.e. the set of means and covariance matrices, and the component weights. We make the assumption that we have a set of training data samples which is assigned to the unit model whose GMM parameters we wish to estimate. In the case of HMM training, such an assignment would be computed with the forward-backward or Viterbi algorithm.

In order to perform model parameter estimation, it is necessary to define a *target criterion* according to which $\boldsymbol{\mu}$, $\boldsymbol{\Sigma}$, and $\mathbf{w}$ are chosen. The standard optimization target, which is the only one which we use for this thesis, is the *maximum likelihood* (ML) criterion: The *likelihood* of the training data is to be maximized. So we define the (logarithmized) *likelihood function* of the training data, given the set of training samples $\mathbf{x} = \{x_1, \dots, x_N\}$ and the GMM parameters $\boldsymbol{\mu}$, $\boldsymbol{\Sigma}$, and $\mathbf{w}$, as follows:

$$\mathcal{L}(\mathbf{x}, \mathbf{w}, \boldsymbol{\mu}, \boldsymbol{\Sigma}) = \sum_{x \in \mathbf{x}} \log \sum_{k} w_k \mathcal{N}(x \,|\, \mu_k, \Sigma_k), \tag{2.4}$$

So the likelihood is computed by evaluating the component Gaussian distributions at each training data vector and then summing over all training data samples. One might furthermore wish to estimate the optimal number K of Gaussian components, but we here assume that K is fixed. Now if there is *just one* Gaussian, i.e. $K = 1$, equation (2.4) can be maximized analytically, the solution is given by

$$\mu_{\mathrm{ML}} = \frac{1}{N}\sum_{n=1}^{N} x_n \quad \text{and} \quad \Sigma_{\mathrm{ML}} = \frac{1}{N}\sum_{n=1}^{N}(x_n - \mu_{\mathrm{ML}})(x_n - \mu_{\mathrm{ML}})^T$$

(for the derivation see any standard textbook, e.g. [Bis07, Chapter 2.3.4]).

Unfortunately, for $K > 1$ there is no closed-form solution for maximizing (2.4) [Bis07, Chapter 9.2]. Instead, an iterative optimization is performed with the *Expectation Maximization* (EM) algorithm, which alternatingly recomputes the feature vector assignments and the Gaussian parameters. We do not give an explicit formula here since we mostly need the Gaussian parameter reestimation in the context of HMM modeling, see section 2.3.5. For details about the EM algorithm for Gaussian mixtures, as well as for a proof of its effectiveness, we refer once more to the excellent textbook [Bis07].

2.3.4 Context Dependency

In the description above, we assumed that for a subphone like H-e, there exists one and only one unit model H-e. This unit model would be used in all words containing the phone [h].

Using such a *context-independent* (CI) structure is certainly possible, since variability of phone realizations is covered by the Gaussian mixture model. However it has been shown in Kai-Fu Lee's doctoral dissertation [Lee88] (we refer to the monograph [Lee89] which Lee published based on his PhD thesis) that the modeling accuracy and, in particular, the recognition accuracy of a speech recognizer improves when *context-dependent* models are used. This means that while the structure of the HMM remains as before, the *emission probabilities*, i.e. the unit models, are changed to reflect not only the current phone, but also the neighboring (context) phones.

Figure 2.13 shows the setup of such an HMM, where a context width of 1 is used, i.e. each phone model depends on its direct left and right neighbors (wider context widths are possible and have been used, too). The notation e.g. *E(H|L)* refers to a unit model for the phone [e] with left context [h] and right context [l]. Note that this GMM still represents *only* the phone [e], *not* the sequence [hel]. Lee reports word-level error reductions of close to 50% relative when using context-dependent modeling [Lee89, Chapter 6.6].

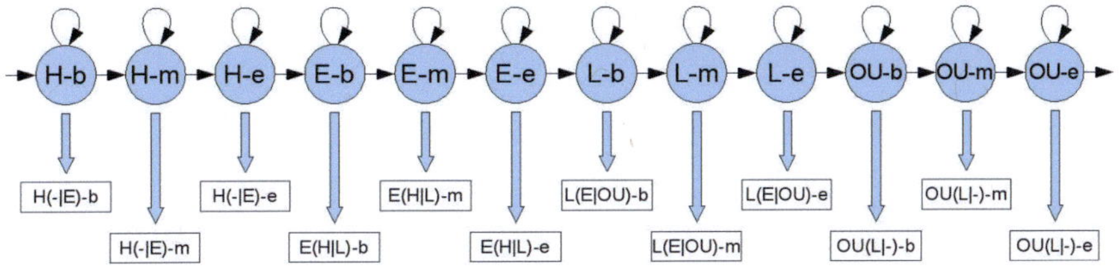

Figure 2.13 – Three-state *Context-Dependent* Phone HMM for the word "Hello", showing the assignment of unit models to HMM states. Each unit model depends on the two neighboring phones as well as on the current phone.

A key challenge in applying context-dependent systems stems from the fact that modeling *each* phone separately depending on its *entire* context would exponentially raise the number of models to be created. This is illustrated with an example computation: Our English-language setup consists of 45 phones plus a special silence phone. Assuming that the non-silence phones are modeled with three substates, we have $3 \cdot 45 + 1 = 136$ models. Using context-dependent modeling with a context width of 1, we get around $45^3 > 90{,}000$ context-dependent phones, yielding more than $270{,}000$ subphone models. The amount of data to reasonably train such a system would be immense: Assume that each unit model is GMM-based with (only) five Gaussian components, and that each Gaussian component requires 100 frames for good estimation (which is not much). Then we need $270{,}000 \cdot 5 \cdot 100$ training data frames, with a frame shift of 10ms, this amounts to $1{,}350{,}000$ seconds, or 375 hours, of required training data. Even if this amount of data is available, it is not clear that the data is sufficiently balanced to allow good training of all GMMs.

According to [Lee89], this problem is solved by creating joint unit models for a group of similar contexts. One could form models by grouping phonetic features: For example, model *E(PLOSIVE |ALVEOLAR)* would be used to represent the phone [e] in words like "tell" or "bed", but not "let" since [l] is not a plosive. This is a *knowledge-based* model structure, since the grouping of contexts is performed according to phonetic knowledge; it is relatively straightforward, but there are several disadvantages:

- It cannot easily be assumed that such a model actually groups contexts which cause similar effects to the center phone.
- There is no guarantee that each model receives enough training data to be estimated reliably.

- It is difficult to adapt the granularity of the context clusters to the available amount of training data.
- Finally, optimizing the context clusters in a practical setting requires a large amount of manual work.

Therefore an automatic clustering is the method of choice. Lee's original algorithm uses a *bottom-up* procedure to merge similar contexts [Lee89, Chapter 6.4], where the similarity between contexts is given by an information-theoretic entropy measure (for background information on information theory and entropy see e.g. [CT91]). After Lee's encouraging results, variations of context-clustering algorithms were rapidly developed. A slightly more recent method, proposed by Bahl and colleagues in 1991 [BdSG+91], remains in widespread use today and is also our method of choice. It uses *phonetic decision trees*, which work on Gaussian Mixture Models. Here, specific models are iteratively created from general ones by *splitting* models based on on phonetic questions: this constitutes a *top-down* approach.

The algorithm works incrementally and creates more and more *specific* models, up to a certain stopping criterion. The basic idea is to go from general models (encompassing many contexts) to specific ones (covering just a few contexts) by splitting models based on a predefined set of phonetic questions. These questions ask about phonetic features of the neighboring phones, examples include: *Is the left-context phone a fricative?* or *Is the right-context phone voiced?*. The model generation algorithm is applied in this thesis in a modified fashion, see section 5.2.2 for a detailed description.

After a phonetic decision tree has been generated, the emission probability for a given HMM state can be computed. We give a concrete example, based on the context decision tree fragment shown in figure 2.14.

The root node represents the end part of the phone [ao] (as in "fall"). If the correct model for the phone [ao] in the word "fall" is to be determined, we start at the root node and answer the questions, based on the phone sequence [f],[ao],[l]: the first question asks "Is the left-context phone (-1) a fricative?". Since the answer is "yes", we continue at node AO(1)-e. The next question asks "Is the right-context phone (+1) voiced?", since [l] is voiced, the answer to the next question is also "yes", so we arrive at node AO(5)-e. This process continues until a leaf node is reached, the leaf node now has an assigned GMM which is used to compute an emission probability. No models are assigned to non-leaf nodes.

The iterative creation of the context decision tree is based on an optimality criterion which in each step considers all possible splits of all existing current leaf nodes and chooses the best available split. The criterion for the choice of the

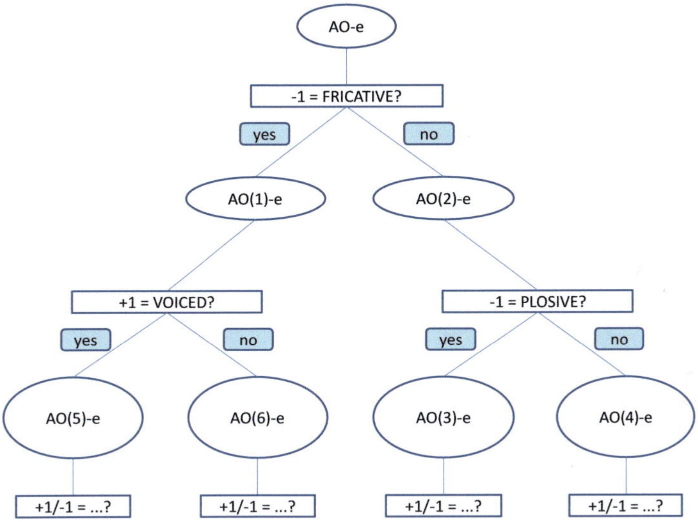

Figure 2.14 – Fragment of a context decision tree in speech recognition

splitting question in each step is the information gain or entropy loss[5] when the split is performed [Lee89, FR97]. The criterion thus reflects the discrepancy between the new phonetic categories which would be created by performing the split: The more they differ, the more benefit is expected from performing the split. The algorithm stops when a predefined number of decision tree leaves has been created, with the additional constraint that the amount of training data per leaf does not fall below a certain threshold. The number of tree leaves is optimized experimentally.

The result of the decision tree algorithm is a set of context-dependent models, created in a data-driven manner to optimize the representation of the observed contexts in the training data.

2.3.5 Bootstrapping and Training

The goal of the training process is the generation of parameters for the Gaussian mixture models (GMM) which form the emission probabilities of the HMM framework. As described above, HMM transition probabilities are not trained.

[5]Note that the terminology regarding the entropy criterion is somewhat nonuniform, [FR97] uses the term "entropy gain", even though the gain is caused by a *loss* of entropy.

The GMM parameters consist of the mixture component weight, mean vector, and covariance matrix for each Gaussian component of the GMMs, as described in section 2.3.3. Furthermore one might wish to determine the optimal number of components for each GMM, and in the context-dependent case, the phonetic decision tree which determines the model structure must be created. We assume that a set of preprocessed transcribed training data is available, where the term *transcribed* means that the textual content of the training data is known (supervised training). This is always the case for the systems considered in this thesis, but in many practical cases, a transcribed training data corpus may not be available. Such cases merit the use of techniques which do not require transcriptions, like *unsupervised adaptation*, which we apply to session-independent systems, see section 8.2.3.

We first consider context-independent modeling. In order to initialize the GMM parameters, an assignment of the feature vectors to the subphone models is required, and it is by no means uncommon to create such an alignment with the help of an already existing speech recognizer. There also exist speech corpora where alignments have been created manually, e.g. the TIMIT corpus [GLF+93], however creating manual time-alignments is an extremely time-consuming process. If alignments exist, initial Gaussian means may be computed with the k-means algorithm (see e.g. [HAH01, Chapter 4.4]) or the merge-and-split algorithm [UNGH00]; the latter automatically estimates the optimal number of components in the Gaussian mixtures. Covariances are normally initialized with the identity matrix.

If no alignment is available, but the amount of training data is large enough, it may be sufficient to initialize all GMM means and covariances uniformly (*flat start*) [You08]. We can *not* use flatstart in the experiments presented in this thesis since the amount of training data has proved to be too small. Instead, we use an acoustic speech recognizer to obtain initial alignments for EMG signals of audibly spoken and whispered speech, see section 4.1.1. For silent speech, a different approach is required, see section 6.3.

The second step deals with finding the optimal parameters for the Gaussians. As described in section 2.3.3, the target function for optimization is the *likelihood function* $\mathcal{L}$, frequently used in logarithmized form for easier computation. In contrast to the usage in section 2.3.3, we incorporate the HMM state (which in the case of context-independent modeling directly corresponds to a unit model) into $\mathcal{L}$. Then $\mathcal{L}$ depends on the following parameters, where the index $m = 1, \ldots, M$ stands for the model (i.e. the GMM), and $k = 1, \ldots, K_m$ stands for the Gaussian component of the GMM m:

- $\mathcal{X} = \{\mathbf{x}_1[t], \ldots, \mathbf{x}_N[t]\}$, the set of all training utterances, where we use t as a (discrete) time parameter, i.e. $t = 1, \ldots, T_n$ for $n = 1, \ldots, N$
- $\mathbf{w} = \{w_{m,k} | m = 1, \ldots, M; k = 1, \ldots, K_m\}$, the set of component weights. It is constrained to have the property that for each model m, $\sum_k w_{m,k} = 1$.
- $\boldsymbol{\mu} = \{\mu_{m,k} | m = 1, \ldots, M; k = 1, \ldots, K_m\}$, the Gaussian means
- $\boldsymbol{\Sigma} = \{\Sigma_{m,k} | m = 1, \ldots, M; k = 1, \ldots, K_m\}$, the Gaussian covariances
- $\mathbf{P} = \{P_1, \ldots, P_N\}$, the possible paths through the HMMs for each training utterance $x_1, \ldots, x_N$. The HMM for an utterance is derived from its transcription. Each P_n is a set of possible paths through the HMM for training utterance x_n, the set of possible paths is determined by the HMM topology. Each *single* path $p \in P_n$ is a sequence of length T_n of model indices.

With these definitions, the log-likelihood function is

$$\mathcal{L}(\mathcal{X}, \mathbf{w}, \boldsymbol{\mu}, \boldsymbol{\Sigma}, \mathbf{P}) = \sum_{\mathbf{x}_n \in \mathcal{X}} \log \sum_{p \in P_n} \sum_{t=1}^{T_n} \sum_{k=1}^{K_{p(t)}} w_{p(t),k} \mathcal{N}(x_n[t] \mid \mu_{p(t),k}, \Sigma_{p(t),k}),$$

i.e. for each training data sample, we evaluate *all* possible paths and then sum over their probabilities. Note that this equation may also be formulated in slightly different ways.

As in the case of single GMMs, the log-likelihood $\mathcal{L}$ cannot be analytically maximized. Fortunately, there exists an efficient algorithm for the optimization of $\mathcal{L}$. It is an instance of the general *Expectation Maximization* (EM) algorithm which we mentioned in section 2.3.3; the update rules for the parameters of the GMM models are known as *Baum-Welch optimization rules.*

We here report the process of HMM training, including the Baum-Welch rules. First assume that we have a "current" set of GMM parameters $\mathbf{w}$, $\boldsymbol{\mu}$, $\boldsymbol{\Sigma}$, they might be initialized using k-means or a similar algorithm. Now two steps are alternatingly performed:

- **Expectation step**: The *assignment probabilities* $\gamma_{m,k}(x)$ are computed. A data sample $x = \mathbf{x}_n[t]$ is by definition *assigned* to one or more Gaussian components of one of more models. This is expressed by the assignment probabilities $\gamma_{m,k}(x)$, where for each x we make the constraint $\sum_{m,k} \gamma_{m,k}(x) = 1$. These assignment probabilities are essentially derived from the probabilities of the paths through the HMM, they can be computed with the forward-backward algorithm or the Viterbi algorithm.

- **Maximization step**: After having fixed the assignment probabilities, we compute new values for $\mathbf{w}$, $\boldsymbol{\mu}$, and $\boldsymbol{\Sigma}$ as follows:

$$\begin{aligned} w_{m,k} &= \frac{N_{m,k}}{N_m}, \\ \mu_{m,k} &= \frac{1}{N_{m,k}} \sum_{\mathbf{x}_n \in \mathcal{X}} \sum_{x \in \mathbf{x}_n} \gamma_{m,k}(x) x, \\ \Sigma_{m,k} &= \frac{1}{N_{m,k}} \sum_{\mathbf{x}_n \in \mathcal{X}} \sum_{x \in \mathbf{x}_n} \gamma_{m,k}(x)(x - \mu_{m,k})(x - \mu_{m,k})^T, \end{aligned} \tag{2.5}$$

  where we have defined $N_{m,k} = \sum_{x \in \mathcal{X}} \gamma_{m,k}(x)$, $N_m = \sum_k N_{m,k}$, and $N = \#\mathcal{X} = \sum_{m,k} N_{m,k}$ (the total amount of training data samples).

We remark that the amount of training data $N_{m,k}$ for any Gaussian component is usually *not* an integer number: Instead it results from the summation of the fractional assignment probabilities of each feature vector to this Gaussian. In other words, training samples are "shared" between Gaussians, each receiving a fraction of this sample according to the assignment probability. For further details about these algorithms, we refer the reader to [Rab89, Bis07].

$\mathcal{L}$ is the probability that the observed samples are *generated* by the underlying probability distributions, i.e. by the Gaussian mixtures. This gives rise to the term *generative modeling* for the parameter estimation method described above. Generative modeling constrasts with *discriminative* methods, where parameters are optimized towards discrimination accuracy. Several such methods exist, including MCE (Minimum Classification Error) training [JCL97], MMIE (Maximum Mutual Information Estimation) training [BBdSM86, WP02], and LMHMM (Large Margin HMM) training [JLL06, SS07]. However, all these methods are computationally expensive, particularly since each sample is used to estimate the assigned models *and* competing models, whereas in generative modeling, each sample only affects the models it is assigned to. In this thesis, only generative modeling is used.

We finally consider the generation of *context-dependent* models. The process of estimating model parameters, described above, does not depend on the exact structure of the models, the only requirement is that we have an assigned model for each HMM state. What we have to do is to *generate* the set of context-dependent models, based on the training data.

This is done as follows. First, a recognizer based on context-independent models is trained. Then the decision tree creation algorithm is run based on this initial model structure, see section 2.3.4, generating a set of context-dependent phone models. Now a *full retraining* of the unit models is performed, based on the new context-dependent structure. We do not give further details on the process of training context-dependent models here, since it large coincides with the generation of *Bundled Phonetic Feature* models, which is described in detail in chapter 5.

2.3.6 Decoding and Language Modeling

Essentially, decoding an unknown speech utterance (assumed to be available in preprocessed form, as usual) requires evaluating HMM models for all possible combinations of words. Then the word combination which yields the highest probability is the recognition *hypothesis*. HMM evaluation could be performed with the forward-backward or Viterbi algorithms.

Of course, if the recognition *vocabulary* (the set of words known to the recognizer) contains more than a small number of words, this approach becomes impractical, or even impossible if the length of an utterance is not known beforehand. Therefore, more versatile methods have to be used.

A very common method uses a *search tree* which is composed from pronunciations of all possible words in the vocabulary. The search tree contains HMM states as nodes and is constructed as a prefix tree, so that words having identical beginnings would be represented by a path in the tree which branches at the phone or state node where the word pronunciations diverge. Initial (root) nodes of the tree correspond to phones which appear at the beginning of words[6], final (leaf) nodes correspond to a full word, which can be determined by following the unique path from a root node to the leaf. The search tree can be visualized as a highly branched HMM. In particular, an emission probability is attached to each tree node.

In most state-of-the-art speech recognizers, decoding is performed time-synchronously, which means that an iteration over frames of the input utterance is performed. In each step, the nodes of the search tree are dynamically tagged with tokens representing partial hypotheses and their probabilities, i.e. each token contains the probability that the assigned tree state is reached at this frame. When a frame is processed, all hypotheses are propagated to their possible successors, and their probabilities are updated using the emission probabilities attached to the tree nodes. Hypotheses which have lower probabilities than competing hypotheses in the same tree node are removed, and more importantly, all hypotheses whose probability falls below a certain (dynamic) threshold are removed, and

[6] strictly speaking, this gives rise not to a single tree, but to a *forest* of multiple trees

only a maximum number of hypotheses is kept at all—this is very important in order to keep the complexity of the algorithm under control.

If a leaf node of the tree is reached, this means that a specific word has been decoded, in the next step, the hypothesis is propagated to the initial nodes, so that sequences of words can be recognized. The algorithm terminates when the input data has been fully processed, then the best existing hypothesis token at any *leaf node* yields the final recognition result. This algorithm is known as *Viterbi Beam Search* [HAH01, Chapter 12], the conceptualization using a search tree and dynamic tokens is called *token passing* [YRT89].

A *language model* contains probabilities for sequences of vocabulary words, *independent* of the observed acoustics. Possible language models include *n-gram* language models, where each sequence of n words receives a probability, and *grammars*, which only allow specific sequences of words. For a detailed discussion of language modeling, we refer to [HAH01, Chapter 11]. In the case of the tree-based decoding described above, language model probabilities are interpolated into the recognition result whenever a word-final (leaf) node is reached [SMFW01].

Due to space constraints, this description of the speech decoding process is kept very brief. For example, we did not mention implementation details like the propagation of word histories in the tokens, dealing with context dependency, and limiting the number of active tokens by pruning those with very low probabilities. Decoding is an active area of research, for further information we refer to the overview in [HAH01, Chapters 12 and 13].

2.4 Dimensionality Reduction by PCA and LDA

The above section introduced feature dimensionality reduction, which is important in the light of the famous concept called "Curse of Dimensionality": When a classifier is trained with relatively high-dimensional input data, and relatively few training samples, *undertraining* may occur. This is a problem for all machine learning algorithms and stems from the underlying assumption that we wish to be able to classify a potentially unlimited set of real-world data, and that we use the training data to gain insight into the properties of this set: This means that we need to learn *general* properties of the data.

All real-world data has got some amount of inherent variability (including artifacts, see section 2.1.3). When undertraining occurs, this inherent variability gains too much influence, so that the learned models represent the specific microstructure of the training data (sometimes exceptionally well), but do not generalize well on unseen data. This means that recognition accuracy on unseen data will degrade, sometimes drastically.

An extreme example of undertraining may be visualized as follows: Assume we intend to train a Gaussian classifier (using just one Gaussian, not a mixture) in a three-dimensional (3D) feature space. We consider the data points belonging to one class: If we have tens, or hundreds of sample feature vectors, it is easy to compute their mean and covariance matrix, and training is finished. If the samples are typical representatives of the data we intend to model (and approximately Gaussian distributed), the resulting classifier should work quite reasonably.

Now assume that only three sample vectors are available for this estimation. Then we can find a *plane* in the feature space which contains all three data points. The resulting Gaussian model is drastically wrong: First, the plane has zero volume in the 3D space, so we model our class as having no volume at all. Second, such a degraded data representation will cause the classifier to malfunction: It will assign zero probability to any data point outside the plane (even if the distance to one of the three training samples is very small), and any data point located on the plane would receive infinite probability. Clearly, such a model fails to yield reasonable results.

Even though this example is extreme, undertraining is a common problem in high-dimensional models, no matter which classifier is used: In all cases, the classifier loses robustness when unseen data is to be processed. Obviously, the allowable input data dimensionality depends on the available amount of training data: If more data is available, higher-dimensional models may be trained. For many practical purposes, including the experiments conducted in this thesis, the amount of training data is fixed, so we need to reduce the data dimensionality in order to allow robust classifier training.

One method of dimensionality reduction was introduced above: *filterbanks* reduce fluctuations in the frequency domain and are applicable to the specific task of generating speech features. However they do not generalize to other types of input data; in particular, EMG data is not processed in the frequency domain (see section 4.1.2), which precludes the application of filterbanks. In this section we explain two common methods of dimensionality reduction which can in principle be applied to all kinds of input data, namely, *Principal Component Analysis (PCA)* and *Linear Discriminant Analysis (LDA)*.

2.4.1 Mathematical Concepts

For the exposition of PCA and LDA, several concepts from linear algebra are required. Here we summarize these notions, without intending to give a full introduction into linear algebra; for background information we refer to standard textbooks. As a prerequisite, we assume that the reader is familiar with the elementary theory of (finite-dimensional) vector spaces and linear maps between them, as well as with inner products (or scalar products, which we denote $\langle x, y\rangle$) and the concept of orthogonality.

Elementary Algebraic Definitions The prototypical finite-dimensional real vector spaces are the spaces $\mathbb{R}^D$ (and their subspaces), with component-wise addition and scalar multiplication. It is easy to show that *any* real finite-dimensional vector space with M dimensions is isomorphic to the $\mathbb{R}^M$, the isomorphism is defined by a *coordinate representation*: Assume that we have an M-dimensional vector space V, and that $B = \{b_1, \ldots, b_M\}$ is a basis of V, i.e. span $(b_1, \ldots, b_M) = V$, and the b_i are linearly independent. Then each element $x \in V$ has got a unique representation $x = \lambda_1 b_1 + \ldots + \lambda_M b_M$ with real numbers λ_i, and we can write x by giving its *coordinates* relative to B:

$$x \cong \begin{pmatrix} \lambda_1 \\ \lambda_2 \\ \vdots \\ \lambda_M \end{pmatrix}.$$

There is an explicit way to compute a coordinate representation in the specific case of an *orthonormal* basis. Assume that $\{b_1, \ldots, b_N\}$ is such a basis, i.e. $\langle b_i, b_j\rangle = 0$ for each pair $i \neq j$, and $||b_i|| = \langle b_i, b_i\rangle = 1$ for all i. Then the coordinate representation of a vector x is given by the real numbers $\lambda_1, \ldots, \lambda_M$ which satisfy $x = \sum_{m=1}^{M} \lambda_m b_m$, and it is easily shown that

$$\lambda_n = \langle x, b_n\rangle. \tag{2.6}$$

We next define *projections*. In general, a projection is a linear map $P : V \to V$ of a vector space into itself, so that the entire image of P remains fixed under P. Projections can be said to "flatten" the input data space, i.e. several dimensions are removed. This is visible in figure 2.15, where two projections are shown: In both cases, the two-dimensional input data is *projected* onto a line A. k is the *direction* of the projection, the right-hand figure shows an *orthogonal* projection, where A and k are orthogonal. Projections can be explicitly defined by basis representations, as follows: Assume that $b_1, \ldots, b_D$ is a basis of the $\mathbb{R}^D$, such

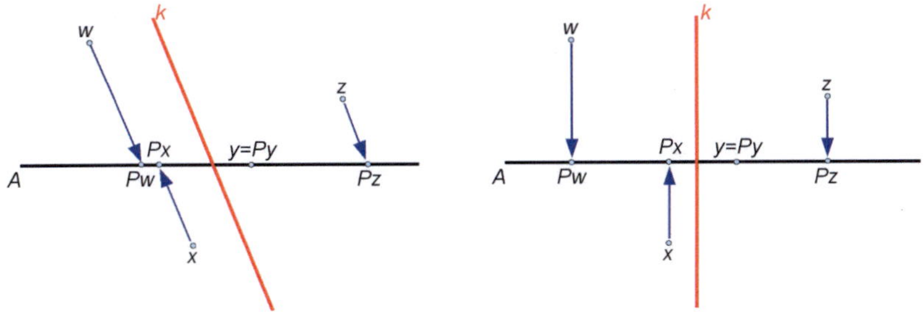

Figure 2.15 – Two examples of projections, which are a specific class of linear mappings which reduce the dimensionality of a linear space. Here two projections P from the two-dimensional space $\mathbb{R}^2$ onto the one-dimensional line $\mathbb{R}^1$ are shown; on the left side, a general projection, on the right side, an *orthogonal* projection.

that $b_1 \dots, b_M$ is a basis of A, and $b_{M+1}, \dots, b_D$ is a basis of k. Then any point $x \in \mathbb{R}^D$ can be written as $x = \sum_{d=1}^{D} \lambda_d b_d$, $\lambda_d \in \mathbb{R}$, and the projection P is explicitly given by

$$P : x = \lambda_1 b_1 + \ldots + \lambda_D b_D \mapsto P(x) = \lambda_1 b_1 + \ldots + \lambda_M b_M, \tag{2.7}$$

so basis vectors belonging to k are omitted. Equations (2.7) and (2.6) finally yield an explicit formula for computing an *orthogonal* projection, which is all we will need for describing the PCA: Assume that A and k are orthogonal, then $\{b_1, \dots, b_D\}$ can be chosen to form an orthonormal basis, and the projection P which projects x to the space span $(b_1, \dots, b_M)$ is given by

$$P(x) = \sum_{d=1}^{M} \langle x, b_d \rangle b_d \cong \begin{pmatrix} \langle x, b_1 \rangle \\ \vdots \\ \langle x, b_M \rangle \end{pmatrix}. \tag{2.8}$$

Projections are at the heart of dimensionality reduction based on linear maps: Indeed, both PCA and LDA consist of a projection of the input data onto a lower-dimensional subspace, and then describing the resulting data *by coordinates* within this subspace. Equation (2.8) shows that in such a case, the coordinate representation of the projection of any $x \in \mathbb{R}^D$ only has $M < D$ dimensions, thus a dimensionality reduction has been achieved.

We now define the PCA algorithm. PCA can be defined in (at least) two equivalent ways, namely, by *variance maximization* or by *projection error minimization.* We introduce PCA by variance maximization and then show that the error minimization formulation yields the same result.

2.4.2 Principal Component Analysis (PCA)

Assume that a set $X = \{x_1, \dots, x_N\} \subset \mathbb{R}^D$ of D-dimensional data samples (i.e. feature vectors) is available, where we assume that the mean of these samples is zero, and where we define Σ_X to be the sample covariance matrix of X. The goal of PCA is to project these feature vectors onto a M-dimensional subspace A of the feature space, where $M < D$. We always assume that we have predetermined a value for M; there are extensions (and even *more* formulations) of the PCA algorithm which allow to determine M from the data [Bis07, Chapter 12.2]. The projected data is to be called $\tilde{X} = \{\tilde{x}_1, \dots, \tilde{x}_N\} \subset \mathbb{R}^M$, and we always understand this to be a coordinate representation with respect to a basis of A, as in equation (2.8).

We require the basis of A to be orthogonal, which is not a restriction, since every subspace of the $\mathbb{R}^D$ has an orthonormal basis. More interestingly, we also require the *projection* to be orthogonal. This can be justified by the fact that out of all possible projections of a point x on a subspace A, the orthogonal projection minimizes the distance (or projection error) $\|x - P(x)\|$.

In order to define the PCA, we need to devise a suitable criterion for optimization. In the one-dimensional case, where the projection space A is a line, the projection is given in coordinates by $P(x) = \langle u_1, x \rangle = u_1^T x$ for a vector u_1 of unit length according to equation (2.8). The criterion is that the *variance* of the projected data, given by

$$\sigma_{\tilde{X}} = \frac{1}{N} \sum_{n=1}^{N} \tilde{x}_n^2 = \frac{1}{N} \sum_{n=1}^{N} u_1^T x_n x_n^T u_1 = u_1^T \Sigma_X u_1, \tag{2.9}$$

is maximized. Note that the projected data still has zero mean. It is not difficult to find a vector u_1 which maximizes this criterion; the standard solution is found by performing a constrained optimization of (2.9) using a Langrange multiplier, see e.g. [Bis07, Chapter 12.1]: u_1 must be an *eigenvector* of Σ_X, namely the one belonging to the *largest* eigenvalue of Σ_X. Below we prove this statement by giving a full justification for the validity of the PCA algorithm even for a multi-dimensional A, the one-dimensional projection is then just a special case.

In order to define PCA in multiple dimensions, i.e. for $M > 1$, we first need to find a criterion which generalizes equation (2.9). We will use the *trace* operator: The trace $\mathrm{Tr}(R)$ of a square matrix $R \in \mathbb{R}^D$ is the sum of its diagonal elements. If R is diagonalizable, $\mathrm{Tr}(R)$ is the sum if the eigenvalues of R (counted with multiplicity), so in particular, there exists the important invariance property that $\mathrm{Tr}(R)$ is invariant under basis changes: $\mathrm{Tr}(S^{-1}RS) = \mathrm{Tr}(R)$ for any invertible matrix S.

Now assume that we project on a multi-dimensional subspace A, which has an orthonormal basis $\{u_1, \ldots, u_M\}$: The projection is then given by

$$P(x) = U^T x \quad \text{with} \quad U = \big(u_1 \mid u_2 \mid \ldots \mid u_M\big) \in \mathbb{R}^{D \times M}. \tag{2.10}$$

Just like in the one-dimensional case, the *covariance matrix* of the projected data is given by $\Sigma_{\tilde{X}} = U^T \Sigma_X U$.

We note one complication in the definition of the multi-dimensional PCA, namely, as long as the optimization criterion only depends on the projection subspace A, it is satisfied by *any* orthonormal basis of A (indeed, even in the one-dimensional case we obviously have two solutions u_1 which maximize (2.9), namely $\pm u_1$). So the basis of A is *not* uniquely defined, and the standard method to determine $u_1, \ldots, u_M$, which we describe below, just chooses the most simple of all possible bases of A: A detail which is skipped even by many standard textbooks (including [Bis07]). However, we will see that as long as all eigenvalues of the data covariance matrix Σ_X are different, the projection subspace A is uniquely determined.

Now we are equipped with the prerequisites to define the maximization criterion for the multi-dimensional PCA. Using the trace operator suggests itself since it does not depend on the particular basis of the projection subspace A, as desired. We choose A to maximize

$$\mathrm{Tr}(\Sigma_{\tilde{X}}) = \mathrm{Tr}(U^T \Sigma_X U), \tag{2.11}$$

where U contains an orthonormal basis of A, as in (2.10). This criterion may also be justified geometrically: The average squared distance of the projected data points $\tilde{x}_1, \ldots, \tilde{x}_N$ from the origin is given by $\sigma_{\tilde{X}}$ in the one-dimensional case, and by $\mathrm{Tr}(\Sigma_{\tilde{X}})$ in the multi-dimensional case (this follows from multiple application of the Theorem of Pythagoras). Thus the multi-dimensional criterion (2.11) and the one-dimensional criterion (2.9) reflect the same geometric property of the projected data.

A direct constrained maximization of (2.11) turns out to be mathematically nontrivial since there is a continuum of solutions. The problem can be solved by imposing additional constraints on the solution, typically it is assumed that the $M+1$-dimensional PCA subspace *includes* the M-dimensional subspace for all $M \in \mathbb{N}$, see e.g. [Bis07]. Yet a solution can also be found without making this assumption, as follows.

Assume that $\lambda_1 \geq \lambda_2 \geq \ldots \geq \lambda_D$ are the sorted eigenvalues of Σ_X[7]. We need to consider all possible subspaces A with dimension M and find (the)

[7] Such an eigenvalue decomposition necessarily exists for any symmetric matrix Σ_X.

one which maximizes $\mathrm{Tr}(\Sigma_{\tilde{X}}) = \mathrm{Tr}(U^T \Sigma_X U)$, where the columns of $U = (u_1 \mid u_2 \mid \ldots \mid u_M)$ contain an orthonormal basis of A.

Below we prove that for any such U,

$$\mathrm{Tr}(\Sigma_{\tilde{X}}) = U^T \Sigma_X U \overset{\ddagger}{\leq} \lambda_1 + \ldots + \lambda_M. \tag{2.12}$$

This implies that any transformation matrix U which yields equality at ‡ solves the M-dimensional PCA problem. In particular, one solution is obtained by choosing $u_1, \ldots, u_M$ as the eigenvectors of Σ_X belonging to the M largest eigenvalues $\lambda_1, \ldots, \lambda_M$: These are easily computed and thus yield the standard solution for the multi-dimensional PCA. Yet it should be clear that any orthogonal transformation of the orthonormal basis of A contained in U yields the same subspace A and thus equally solves the problem. We obtain the solution to the one-dimensional projection (u_1 must be an eigenvector with eigenvalue λ_1) as a special case, and we also see that the subspace A is uniquely defined if and only if $\lambda_M > \lambda_{M+1}$.

Proof of inequality (2.12):
Let $\lambda_1 \geq \lambda_2 \geq \ldots \geq \lambda_D$ the sorted eigenvalues of Σ_X. We can write them as the diagonal elements of a matrix Λ:

$$\Lambda = \begin{pmatrix} \lambda_1 & 0 & \ldots & 0 \\ 0 & \lambda_2 & \ldots & 0 \\ \vdots & \vdots & \ddots & \vdots \\ 0 & 0 & \ldots & \lambda_D \end{pmatrix},$$

then there is an orthogonal matrix V (i.e. a matrix whose rows and columns form an orthonormal basis of $\mathbb{R}^D$), such that $\Sigma_X = V^T \Lambda V$.

Assume that $\Sigma_{\tilde{X}} = U^T \Sigma_X U$. Then for $W = VU = ((w_{ij})) \in \mathbb{R}^{D \times M}$, it holds that $\Sigma_{\tilde{X}} = W^T \Lambda W$, and thus for the j-th diagonal element d_j of $\Sigma_{\tilde{X}}$, we have $d_j = \sum_{i=1}^{D} w_{ij}^2 \lambda_i$, $1 \leq j \leq M$. Consequently,

$$\mathrm{Tr}(\Sigma_{\tilde{X}}) = \sum_{j=1}^{M} d_j = \sum_{j=1}^{M} \left(\sum_{i=1}^{D} w_{ij}^2 \lambda_i \right) = \sum_{i=1}^{D} \left(\sum_{j=1}^{M} w_{ij}^2 \right) \lambda_i = \sum_{i=1}^{D} \alpha_i \lambda_i \tag{2.13}$$

with $\alpha_i = \sum_{j=1}^{M} w_{ij}^2$. The *columns* of $W \in \mathbb{R}^{D \times M}$ contain an orthonormal basis of a subspace of $\mathbb{R}^D$, thus their squared norm is one, and similarly, the squared

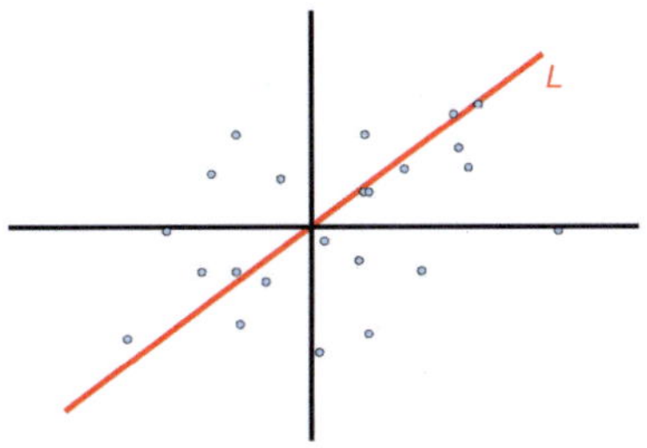

Figure 2.16 – PCA for a one-dimensional projection space. The line L is in the direction of maximal variance.

norm of the *rows* of W must be less or equal one:

$$\begin{aligned} \sum_{i=1}^{D} w_{ij}^2 &= 1 \quad \text{for all } j \in \{1, \ldots, M\} \\ \sum_{j=1}^{M} w_{ij}^2 &\leq 1 \quad \text{for all } i \in \{1, \ldots, D\}. \end{aligned} \tag{2.14}$$

The first part of (2.14) implies

$$\sum_{i=1}^{D} \sum_{j=1}^{M} w_{ij}^2 = M. \tag{2.15}$$

From equations (2.13) – (2.15) we obtain $\text{Tr}(\Sigma_{\tilde{X}}) = \sum_{i=1}^{D} \alpha_i \lambda_i$ with $0 \leq \alpha_i \leq 1$ and $\sum_{i=1}^{D} \alpha_i = M$, and since the λ_i are sorted by decreasing value, we immediately conclude that $\text{Tr}(\Sigma_{\tilde{X}}) \leq \lambda_1 + \ldots + \lambda_M$, which is what we intended to show. ■

Thus, we have fully defined the Principal Component Analysis (PCA), using the variance maximization criterion (2.11): The PCA projection of X on an M-dimensional subspace is obtained by choosing the subspace spanned by the M eigenvectors of Σ_X with the M highest eigenvalues. An example for $M = 1$ is shown in figure 2.16. We see that given a set of D-dimensional data, finding the PCA projection amounts to computing the second-order statistics of the input data, and finding the eigenvectors of a $D \times D$-matrix. This may be done using standard numerical methods and is very efficient, even for high-dimensional data.

Finally, it is easy to show that PCA can also be defined in a second way, yielding the same result. We again fix the following prerequisites: We have a set

$X = \{x_1, \ldots, x_N\}$ of D-dimensional input data with zero mean, and we search a projection onto an M-dimensional subspace. The goal is now to *minimize the squared projection error*, given by

$$E(U, X) = \sum_{n=1}^{N} \|x_n - P(x_n)\|^2, \tag{2.16}$$

where $P(x) = U^T x$ is the projection to be found. $E(U, X)$ measures the error which is made when we replace all x_n with $P(x_n)$.

Above, we remarked that it suffices to consider orthogonal projections. So assume that we have an orthonormal basis $b_1, \ldots, b_M$ of a projection subspace, which is extended to an orthonormal basis of the $\mathbb{R}^D$ by the vectors $b_{M+1}, \ldots, b_D$. Let $U = \left(b_1 \mid \ldots \mid b_M\right)$, and similarly $V = \left(b_{M+1} \mid \ldots \mid b_D\right)$. Then with a geometric argument similar to the one used to justify the multi-dimensional PCA criterion, it can be shown that $\mathrm{Tr}(V^T \Sigma_X V)$ is the average squared distance of the data points x_n to the projection subspace:

$$E(U, X) = \mathrm{Tr}(V^T \Sigma_X V).$$

Since $b_1, \ldots, b_D$ is a basis of the whole $\mathbb{R}^D$, it is also clear that $\mathrm{Tr}(U^T \Sigma_X U) + \mathrm{Tr}(V^T \Sigma_X V) = \mathrm{Tr}(\Sigma_X)$, which is a constant. Now one immediately concludes that minimizing $E(U, X) = \mathrm{Tr}(V^T \Sigma_X V)$ amounts to maximizing $\mathrm{Tr}(U^T \Sigma_X U)$. This was our original variance maximization criterion, so we have shown that the criteria (2.16) and (2.11) yield the same result.

2.4.3 Linear Discriminant Analysis

Finally we discuss *Linear Discriminant Analysis (LDA)* as a dimensionality reduction tool, using [Bis07, Chapter 4.1.4] as our main reference. In contrast to PCA, the central assumption is now that we have *class assignments* for all our data points, and that the goal of dimensionality reduction is finding a low-dimensional data representation for training a classifier.

A typical example of LDA is shown in figure 2.17. There are two classes of data points, and we intend to find a projection on a one-dimensional line. The PCA subspace is shown as a red line, and it is clear that it is optimal for *representing* the data points, but suboptimal for *classifying* them. The figure also shows a better solution: Projecting the samples on the green “LDA” line would yield fully separated classes even in one dimension.

Creating an exact algorithm to compute such a projection is somewhat more involved than doing PCA, in particular, we need to define a suitable optimization

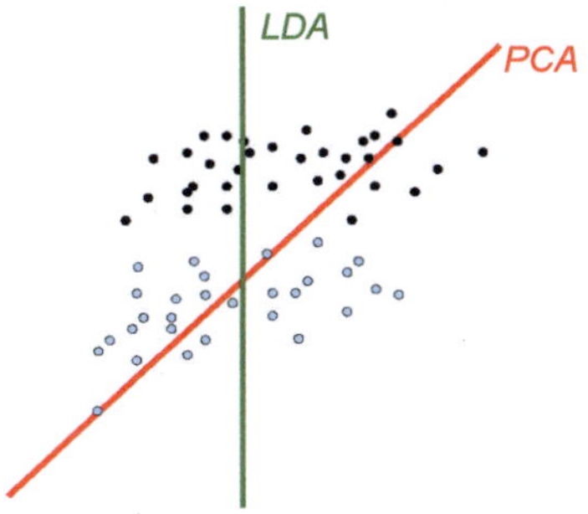

Figure 2.17 – Linear discriminant analysis: Assume that we have a dataset with known class assignments (depicted by light and dark points), and that we intend to train a classifier based on dimensionality-reduced features. Then the PCA projection (red line) may not be optimal: It would cause a substantial overlap between classes. The problem is solved by the LDA projection (green line).

criterion. Exact class separability cannot be the criterion of choice, in particular since it is not usually achievable: In practice, classes overlap even without dimensionality reduction. Also, a criterion depending on single data points violating a class boundary would be extremely sensitive to outliers, and even a perfect solution might be inadequate since we later on wish to classify *unseen* data.

As for the PCA, instead of looking at single data points we consider statistical properties of the classes as a whole. In order to give an intuitive introduction to LDA, we consider the most simple case: We have two data sets $Y = \{y_1, \ldots, y_{N_Y}\}$ and $Z = \{z_1, \ldots, z_{N_Z}\}$ for which an optimally separating projection is to be found, and we limit the projection subspace to one dimension, i.e. a line. As for the PCA, we assume that the *full* set of samples $X = Y \cup Z$ has zero mean ($\mu_X = 0$): Then we will be able to find a projection on a subspace going through the origin.

The projection has the form

$$P(x) = w^T x = \langle w, x \rangle$$

for a direction vector w and any sample $x \in X$. In order to find w, we make the following definitions:

- The class-wise means are named μ_Y resp. μ_Z. Note that they are not required to be zero (only the *entire* data set must have zero mean). Also, the class-wise covariance matrices are named Σ_Y and Σ_Z. N_Y and N_Z are the number of elements per class, and $N = N_Y + N_Z$.

- The *total scatter* Σ_T is the covariance matrix of the entire data set.
- The *between scatter* Σ_B is the covariance matrix of the *class means*, each weighted with the number of elements per class:

$$\Sigma_B = \frac{1}{N}(N_Y \mu_Y + N_Z \mu_Z)$$

(remember that we assumed that the mean of the entire data set is zero: Otherwise we would have to replace μ_Y by $\mu_Y - \mu_X$, and μ_Z by $\mu_Z - \mu_X$).

- The *within scatter* is the average of the within-class covariance matrices, again weighted with the number of elements per class:

$$\Sigma_W = \frac{1}{N}(N_Y \Sigma_Y + N_Z \Sigma_Z).$$

The scatter matrices then satisfy the important property $\Sigma_T = \Sigma_W + \Sigma_B$.

The LDA criterion (also known as *Fisher criterion*) is to simultaneously *maximize* the between scatter and *minimize* the within scatter: This means that we find a projection which pushes the classes far apart, but also makes each class as compact as possible. From figure 2.17, one can see that in direction of the "LDA" line, this criterion is indeed satisfied.

In order to mathematically formulate the LDA criterion, we need to compute the scatters of the *projected* data, which works exactly as in equation (2.9): The between scatter of the projected data is the scalar value $w^T \Sigma_B w$, the within scatter of the projected data is similarly computed as $w^T \Sigma_W w$. Now the fisher criterion can be written as

$$w = \arg\max_{\hat{w}} J(\hat{w}) = \arg\max_{\hat{w}} \frac{\hat{w}^T \Sigma_B \hat{w}}{\hat{w}^T \Sigma_W \hat{w}}.$$

A maximum can be found by solving a generalized eigenvalue problem for Σ_B and Σ_W, i.e. w is computed to solve the expression

$$\Sigma_B \cdot w = \Sigma_W \cdot w \cdot \delta \tag{2.17}$$

with a scalar δ, and w is chosen so that δ is maximized.

We can legitimately ask whether such a w exists, and what its properties are. In case Σ_W is invertible, we can left-multiply equation (2.17) by Σ_W^{-1} and obtain $(\Sigma_W^{-1}\Sigma_B)w = \delta w$, so we see that w is just an eigenvector of $\Sigma_w^{-1}\Sigma_B$, which always exists since $\Sigma_W^{-1}\Sigma_B$ is a symmetric matrix. However, if Σ_W is *not* invertible, $J(w)$ is undefined for a w chosen to be an eigenvector of Σ_W with zero eigenvalue. In terms of the input data, such a w indicates a direction in which all classes have

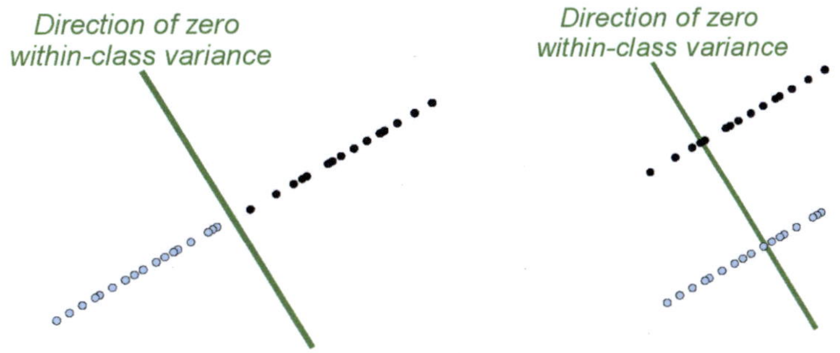

Figure 2.18 – Two examples where the within-class scatter is zero along one direction. In the first case (left), projecting on that direction would yield no discrimination at all, in the second case (right), the direction yields excellent classification.

zero variance, as shown in figure 2.18: It might be acceptable to project on such a direction, or it might yield no discrimination at all. The criterion $J(w)$ fails to distinguish such cases.

Such a situation may emerge in fields like image processing, where one might wish to process a few hundred images each having tens of thousands of pixels. In our case, eigenvalues are rarely *exactly* zero, but very *small* eigenvalues frequently occur when a small amount of high-dimensional input data is to be processed. Even then, the maximization of $J(w)$ becomes numerically unstable. This problem stems from the division in the definition of $J(w)$ (in particular, PCA does not suffer from this issue), and it has been observed in practical applications, see e.g. [QZH09]. A standard solution is *regularization* [Fri89]: In its simplest form, the within-scatter matrix Σ_W is replaced by $\Sigma_W + \beta I$, where I is the identity matrix, and $\beta > 0$ is a regularization parameter. $\Sigma_W + \beta I$ is a regular matrix: Since Σ_W is a covariance matrix, it cannot have negative eigenvalues, thus all eigenvalues of $\Sigma_W + \beta I$ must be strictly positive. For our high-dimensional array system, presented in chapter 7, we observed good results using this method, even with varying parameters β.

Finally, we define the multidimensional LDA. Here we assume that the set of samples is devided into K classes, and that we wish to project the input data on an M-dimensional subspace. Now the projection takes the form $P(x) = W^T x$ for a $M \times D$ matrix W. The definitions of the total scatter, between scatter, and within scatter are directly generalized to the multidimensional case, and we just need a new maximization criterion. A standard choice [Fuk90] is

$$J(W) = \mathrm{Tr}((W^T \Sigma_W W)^{-1}(W^T \Sigma_B W)), \tag{2.18}$$

which is justified by similar arguments as the multi-dimensional PCA criterion. This equation is maximized by solving a generalized eigenvalue problem, like in the one-dimensional case [Fuk90]. We remark that optimizing the criterion (2.18) yields a subspace of at most $K-1$ dimensions (i.e. one dimension less than there are sample classes), since the rank of Σ_B is at most $K-1$. So the projection subspace dimensionality M must be smaller than the number of classes.

We finally note that there are several variations of the LDA criterion, for example, the total scatter can replace the within scatter due to the relation $\Sigma_T = \Sigma_W + \Sigma_B$. We implemented several such variations, but on our EMG data we never found any substantial difference between these approaches.

Chapter 3

Experimental Setup and Corpus

This chapter describes the two EMG recording setups which are used in this thesis, and gives statistics about the recorded data corpora. The setups differ in the EMG capturing: For the majority of the experiments, we use a setup based on 6 EMG channels, derived at carefully selected positions in the face. The most recent experiments are based on electrode arrays, which are electrode grids with multiple measuring points. Based on the two setups, three data corpora have been used for experiments, two of which were created as part of this thesis.

3.1 The Cognitive Systems Lab EMG Acquisition System

This section deals with EMG signal capturing for the specific purpose of recording speech-related muscle activity. Two setups are presented, namely a six-channel setup based on single electrodes, and a setup based on *electrode arrays* which was developed as part of this thesis.

Figure 3.1 shows the major muscles of the human face. Not all of these muscles are easily captured by electromyography: The respective muscle should be located close to the skin surface, and an electrode placed above the muscle should not interfere with the process of speaking. Additional constraints are imposed by the recording hardware, in particular, for the recordings with our single-electrode setup, only six to eight EMG channels could be recorded. However, each EMG channel is expected to capture signals from different nearby muscles.

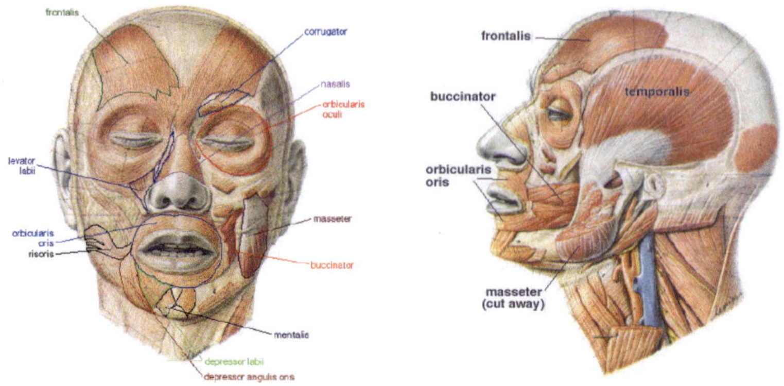

Figure 3.1 – Major muscles of the human head and face (from `http://www.yorku.ca/earmstro/`, used with permission)

Due to the limited number of EMG channels, we do not assume that our recording setup captures *all* speech-related activity. While it is attempted to cover the most important muscles, the resulting data is classified *statistically* without endeavoring to perform a decomposition of the recorded signals into their constituting components (a nontrivial problem even with optimal muscle coverage).

The following sections describe the two recording setups in detail.

3.1.1 Single-Electrode Setup

The majority of the experiments in this thesis is based on a six-channel "single-electrode" setup, which was developed in 2005 by L. Maier-Hein [MH05a]. We use surface electrodes with a circular recording area having a diameter of 4 mm: given the finely grained motor unit control of the facial muscles, it is clear that any such electrode will pick up signals of plenty of motor units and even of different muscles. The electrodes are standard Ag/AgCl electrodes. Conductive gel is applied to the electrode/skin junction in order to reduce the contact impedance. Two corpora were recorded with this setup, namely the EMG-PIT corpus and the EMG-UKA corpus, see section 3.2.

The optimal setup from [MH05a] is shown in figure 3.2: It covers a large set of facial muscles (see figure 3.1), while limiting the number of channels to six. This is a technical limitation of the recording hardware, but on the other hand, the smaller the number of EMG electrodes, the less discomfort to the user, and the shorter the preparation time. This setup has proved easy-to-use and stable,

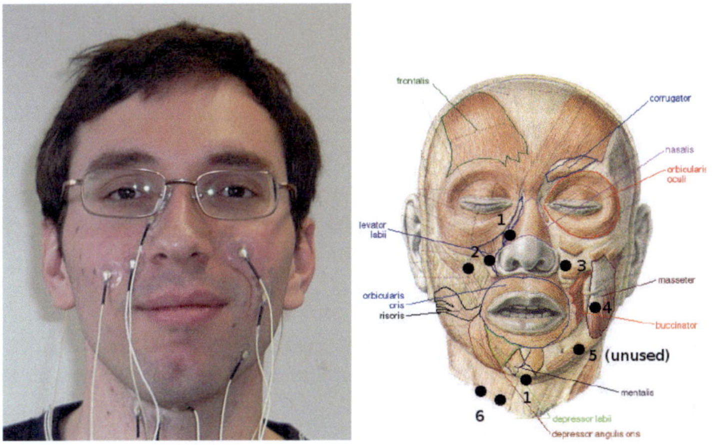

Figure 3.2 – Electrode positioning for the single-electrode setup (muscle chart adapted from `http://www.yorku.ca/earmstro/`, with permission)

therefore is has been used ever since its creation, including for the PhD thesis of S. Jou [Jou08].

The six recorded EMG channels capture activity from the levator anguli oris (channels 2, 3), the zygomaticus major (channels 2, 3), the platysma (channels 4, 5) the depressor anguli oris (channel 5), the anterior belly of the digastric (channel 1) and the tongue (channel 1, 6) [MHMSW05, UCL02]. EMG channels 2 and 6 use bipolar derivation, the other channels are derived unipolarly, with a reference electrode on the nose (channel 1) respectively two connected reference electrodes behind the ears (channels 3, 4, 5). Note that in our experiments, we follow [JSW$^+$06] in removing channel 5, which tends to yield unstable and artifact-prone signals.

The relationship between the facial muscles, the articulatory gestures these muscles generate, and the produced sounds is well-researched, albeit quite intricate. Table 3.1, a reproduction of table 2.2 from the original study by L. Maier-Hein [MH05a], summarizes the roles of the major articulatory muscles in the movement of the articulators. The relationship between the articulators and the production of sounds has been described in sections 2.2.1 and 2.2.2, we do not repeat the details here: In general, the sound of vowels is mostly determined by the position of the tongue and the lips, whereas consonants articulation is characterized by an obstruction in the vocal tract which frequently requires the interplay of various articulators.

Muscle Name	Function
Orbicularis oris	On contraction, this muscle adducts the lips by drawing the lower lip up and the upper lip down, probably in conjunction with some of the other facial muscles. It may also pull the lips against the teeth. This muscle can also round the lips by its sphincter action.
Zygomaticus major	Raises upper lip for [f] along with the muscles that raise the angles of the mouth. On contraction, this muscle draws the angle of the mouth upward and laterally. The upward movement probably works with levator anguli oris to achieve the raised upper lip in labiodental fricatives. The lateral movement may be used in the production of [s].
Levator Anguli Oris	This muscle draws the corner of the mouth upwards and, because of the fibers that insert into the lower lip, may assist in closing the mouth by drawing the lower lip up, for the closure phase in bilabial consonants.
Depressor Anguli Oris	This muscle depresses the angles of the lips. This action may work with depressor labii inferioris to prevent the mouth from closing entirely when spreading for vowels like [i] and [e]. Because of the fibers that insert in the upper lip, this muscle may also aid in compressing lips by drawing the upper lip down.
Platysma	The platysma can aid depressor anguli oris and depressor labii inferioris to draw down and laterally the angles of the mouth.
Anterior Belly of the Digastric	The function of this muscle is to draw the hyoid bone up and forward. It also serves to bring the tongue forward and upward for alveolar and high front vowel articulations. In pulling up the hyoid bone, it may also pull up the larynx thereby tensing the stretching the vocal cords and raising the pitch. If the hyoid bone is fixed, the anterior belly of the digastric can serve to lower the jaw in conjunction with the geniohyoid, mylohyoid and lateral pterygoid muscles.

Table 3.1 – Functionality of the muscles involved in speech production (taken from [MH05a])

When audible or whispered speech are recorded, the audio signal is simultaneously captured with a standard close-talking headset microphone connected to a USB soundcard; we use the term *parallel* acoustic data to refer to these recordings. Wearing the headset does not interfere with the EMG electrodes. The EMG signal is delayed by 50 ms so that it aligns with the audio signal, this *anticipatory effect* of the EMG signal was investigated in detail in [JSW+06], following earlier work in [CEHL02]. Note that this effect is *not* related to the recording hardware or setup, but is a genuine property of the myoelectric signal which has been reported in literature [CK79]. It is also used in other contexts, for example, the DIVA model of articulation [GGT06], which is described in detail in section 6.1, uses a movement onset latency of 42 ms with respect to the neuromuscular activation.

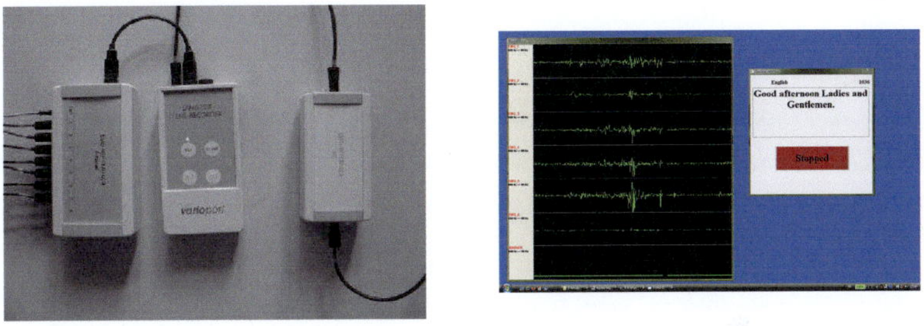

Figure 3.3 – EMG Recorder and Recording Software screenshot for the single-channel electrode setup (left picture from [MH05a])

EMG recordings are performed with the *Varioport* biosignal recorder (Becker Meditec, Germany), which is shown in the left-hand part of figure 3.3. From left to right, one can see the EMG amplifier, the recorder, and an electrical insulation device which separates the electrical currents of the recorder and the connected PC or laptop. The recorder is battery-powered. Technical specifications of this system include an amplification factor of 1170, 16 bits A/D conversion, a resolution of 0.033 microvolts per bit, and a frequency range of 0.9-295 Hz. Sampling is performed with a 600 Hz sampling rate, which is slightly lower than suggested in [FC86], but nonetheless captures most EMG activity measurable at the skin surface; the sampling rate is limited by the serial connection between the EMG recorder and the controlling PC, among other factors.

We note that two different EMG amplifiers were used for recordings: Recordings for the EMG-PIT corpus used an 8-channel amplifier, and recordings for the EMG-UKA corpus used a (newer) 6-channel amplifier. These two amplifiers exhibit different analog filter characteristics, which has got a visible impact on the presence of artifacts in the recorded signal. In particular, low-frequency artifacts

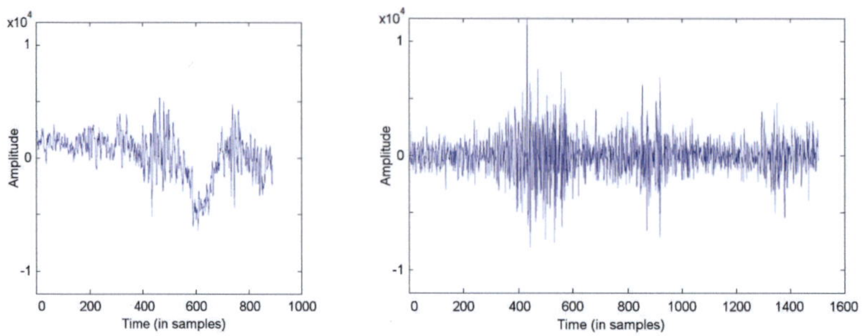

Figure 3.4 – Example for EMG signals (single-electrode setup, channel 1) of the utterance "We can do it", recorded with two different EMG amplifiers. The left signal (from the EMG-PIT corpus, recorded with the 8-channel amplifier) exhibits substantially more low-frequency artifacts than the right-hand signal (from the EMG-UKA corpus, recorded with the 6-channel amplifier).

are substantially more prevalent in the EMG-PIT corpus than in the EMG-UKA corpus. Example signals of the utterance "We can do it" are shown in figure 3.4.

Besides the EMG input, the Varioport recorder allows the capturing of up to two auxiliary channels, one of which is used for hardware synchronization of the recorded EMG signal and acoustic signal: At the beginning of the recording of each utterance, a synchronization signal for the EMG and acoustic data is created by the recording software and made available at the parallel port of the recording PC. The parallel port is connected to one auxiliary channel of the Varioport recorder, so that the synchronization signal is recorded together with the EMG data; note that we use an electrical insulation device for this connection, too. For synchronization with the audio data, we use stereo (i.e. two-channel) recording: The first stereo channel contains the actual acoustic signal, the second channel contains the synchronization signal.

For recording control, the in-house software *UKA EEG/EMG Studio* developed by C. Mayer et al. [May] is used. The user interface is shown in the right-hand part of figure 3.3: The six recorded EMG channels are displayed in real-time, so that artifacts can be detected and, hence, avoided during the recording process. The subject sees the prompt window on the right side, in order to start a recording, the red button must be pressed. While the button remains pressed, recording of the EMG signal takes place. The control window, containing settings for the experiment supervisor, is not shown.

The recorded EMG and acoustic data, including the synchronization signal, is saved on the hard disk in an uncompressed format. At the end of a session, a text file containing information about the recorded utterances, including a transcription of their content, is created.

3.1.2 Electrode Array Setup

Electrode Arrays are grid structures with multiple measuring points for bioelectric signals. They may be as small as 2x2 electrodes [dLAW$^+$06], but can also be much larger, e.g. [YZXL13] uses an array with $16 \times 6 = 96$ channels. The multi-channel high-density EMG measurements which are made possible by EMG arrays offer possibilities for artifact reduction, feature extraction, and signal analysis, which we discuss in detail in section 7. Therefore, one part of this thesis has been the creation of a facial EMG recording setup which makes use of EMG array technology, and the subsequent recording of a data corpus of multi-channel EMG recordings of speech. We first reported on this new setup in [WSJS13].

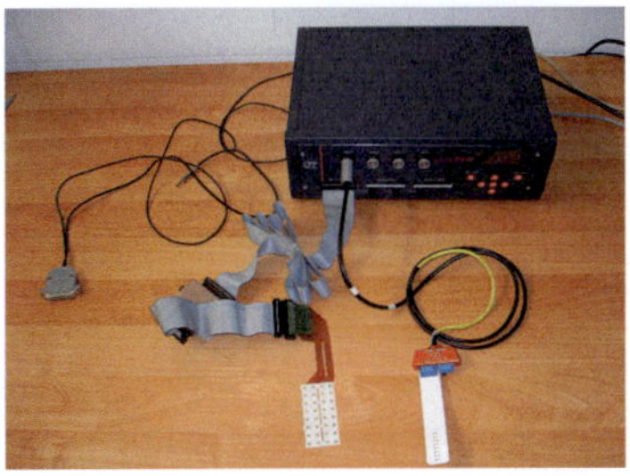

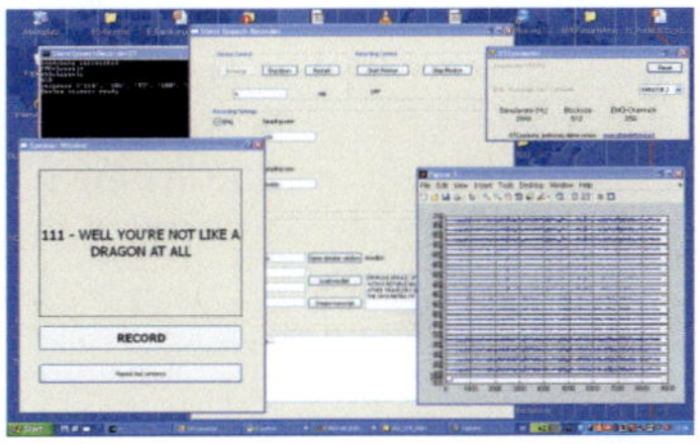

Figure 3.5 – EMG Recorder and Recording Software screenshot for the electrode array setup

For this purpose, the multi-channel EMG amplifier *EMG-USB2* was purchased from OT Bioelettronica, Italy (`http://www.otbioelettronica.it`), together with a set of matching arrays. The amplifier supports the capturing of up to 256 channels; further technical specifications include an amplification factor of up to 10000 and a maximum sampling rate of 10240 Hz, a configurable bandwidth between 3 Hz and 4400 Hz, and 12 bit A/D conversion [OT]. A *DRL circuit* [WW83] is used to reduce common mode voltage noise. In our experiments, we used a sampling rate of 2048 Hz.

The acoustic signal is simultaneously recorded with a close-talking microphone for the audible and whispered speaking modes, yielding parallel acoustic and EMG data. Synchronization of the EMG and acoustic signals is performed as for the single-electrode setup: the EMG amplifier allows to record up to 16 non-amplified auxiliary channels, one of which is used for the synchronization signal;

the acoustic data contains the synchronization signal in the second stereo channel. The EMG signal is delayed by 50 ms to align with the audio signal, as in the single-electrode setup.

The left-hand part of figure 3.5 shows the EMG-USB2 amplifier, together with some instrumentation. It can be seen that in contrast to the Varioport device, the EMG-USB2 amplifier is a non-portable, "tabletop" device.

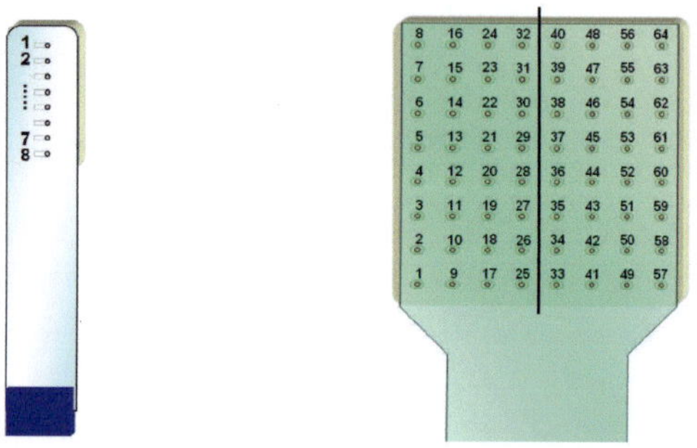

Figure 3.6 – The EMG arrays which were used in this study. The left-hand array has 8 EMG channels with a distance of 5 mm, the right-hand array has $8 \times 8 = 64$ channels with a distance of 1 cm in both directions. The 64-channel array was cropped to 4×8 electrodes, as indicated by the black line. Images from [Sch11].

Figure 3.6 shows the two types of EMG arrays which were used for the experiments presented in this thesis. We use an 8-channel array with 5 mm IED (inter-electrode distance) and a 64-channel array with eight rows of eight electrodes with 1 cm IED. The 64-channel array is user-configurable and can be flexibly cropped according to the experimental requirements: for facial EMG recordings, we cut off the right half of the array, so that $4 \times 8 = 32$ electrodes remain. The EMG arrays require electrolyte gel, just like the classical electrodes described in section 3.1.1, however the manufactorer provides electrolyte gel in form of a *cream*—our subjects found this much more comfortable than standard medical-issue electrode gel.

The EMG channels are arranged sequentially, so that both unipolar and bipolar recordings are possible: For unipolar recordings, a ground electrode is placed on the subject's neck, for bipolar recordings, the difference of each pair of channels with consecutive numbers is computed. This means that e.g. for the eight-channel array, we obtain seven bipolar EMG signals, namely from the differences $2-1, 3-2, ..., 8-7$. Similarly, for the (full) 64-channel array, one obtains 56 bipolar EMG signals, bipolar signals stemming from distant electrode pairs (like $9-8$, $17-16$, etc., see figure 3.6), these signals are considered invalid.

Speaking mode	Average data length per session, in seconds			sessions / speakers
	Train	Test	Total	
Development ("pilot") set				
audible EMG	180	52	232	28/14
silent EMG	184	53	237	27/14
Total amount of data: 3:35 hours				
Evaluation ("main") set				
audible EMG	197	57	254	62/62
silent EMG	186	54	240	62/62
Total amount of data: 8:30 hours				

Table 3.2 – EMG-PIT data corpus

Recordings with the array-based setup were controlled using the *OT Biolab* software delivered with the EMG-USB2 amplifier. OT Biolab offers real-time visualization of a large number of recorded channels, and the signal is made available at a system socket for reading by the recording software. For recording, we used the in-house software BiosignalsStudio [HPA+10], a flexible, modular toolbox for biosignal recording with various setups and devices. We programmed a custom interface for our recordings, similar to the interface used for the single-electrode setup, which is shown in the right-hand part of figure 3.5.

3.2 Data Corpora

3.2.1 The EMG-PIT Data Corpus

The *EMG-PIT* corpus was cooperatively recorded by Carnegie Mellon University, Pittsburgh, PA, USA, and the Voice Lab of the University of Pittsburgh. The responsible experimenters were S. Jou and M. Dietrich, who recorded the EMG data as part of their respective PhD theses [Jou08, Die08].

The EMG-PIT corpus uses the single-electrode setup described in section 3.1.1; its key feature is a large number of recorded speakers: Altogether, the corpus comprises 76 speakers. This allows experiments on speaker-independent recognition, see section 8.1.2. All subjects were female native speakers of English, aged 18 – 35 years.

The EMG-PIT corpus consists of two parts, the *pilot* part and the *main* part. For the pilot part, each subject was recorded twice, for the main part, each subject was recorded only once. The recordings were part of a larger study, as detailed in [Die08], however the data which is used in this thesis was always recorded as a consecutive block (this is relevant for assuring a constant data quality since during long-term EMG recording, the electrode-skin contact and hence the EMG signal may vary substantially).

The subjects read phonetically balanced sentences in a quiet room and a controlled setting (recognizing conversational, unplanned speech using EMG is beyond the scope of this thesis). The sentence lists were in English language, they were taken from the Broadcast News domain, a well-researched standard domain in acoustic speech recognition. Each sentence list consisted of 50 sentences, divided into a batch of 10 *BASE* sentences which were identical for all speakers and all sessions, and one batch of 40 *SPEC* sentences, which varied across sessions. In each session these sentences were recorded twice, once for each speaking mode, i.e. for audible speech and for silent speech. For brevity, we call the EMG signals from these parts *audible EMG*, and *silent EMG*, respectively. The sentence sets were identical for both speaking modes, so that the database covers both speaking modes with parallel utterances. The total of 50 BASE and SPEC utterances in each part were recorded in random order. For all experiments, the SPEC sentences are used as training data, and the BASE sentences are used as test data. Furthermore, we set the main part of the EMG-PIT corpus aside, so that it could be used as an evaluation set. The EMG-PIT corpus is summarized in table 3.2, note that in one session, the silent recordings were damaged and had to be removed.

3.2.2 The EMG-UKA Data Corpus

The EMG-UKA corpus was recorded during the creation of this thesis and constitutes an integral part of it. The main goals which the EMG-UKA corpus addresses were obtaining a large number of recording session from *one* speaker, and recording EMG data of whispered speech in addition to audible and silent speech. Therefore, the full EMG-UKA corpus has three non-disjoint subsets: The *multi-session subset*, which is intended for experiments on session independency and session adaptation (see chapter 8), the *multi-mode subset*, which contains recordings of all three speaking modes and is used for multi-mode and cross-mode recognition (see chapter 6), and the *single-session subset*, which consists of all audible EMG recording sessions of the entire corpus. The recording setup for this corpus was the exact same single-electrode setup as was used for the EMG-PIT corpus, however the EMG amplifier was different, see section 3.1.1.

Speaking mode	Average data length per session, in seconds Train	Test	Total	sessions / speakers
Single-Session subset				
audible EMG	147	42	189	61/8
Total amount of data: 3:12 hours				
Multi-mode subset				
audible EMG	156	44	200	30/8
whispered EMG	160	45	205	
silent EMG	158	44	202	
Total amount of data: 5:04 hours				
Multi-session subset				
audible EMG	142	41	183	48/2
Total amount of data: 2:26 hours				
Entire EMG-UKA corpus: 6:35 hours				

Table 3.3 – EMG-UKA data corpus. Note that the subsets are *not* disjoint.

The recording protocol of the EMG-UKA corpus follows the EMG-PIT corpus to ensure compatibility. In particular, we used the same English sentence lists as were used for recording the EMG-PIT corpus. The subjects did *not* speak English natively, however we made sure that the subject's knowledge of English pronunciation was sufficiently good for the intended purpose of speech recognition, and during the recordings, the supervisor corrected major pronunciation mistakes. The 50 sentences per recording session were recorded either once, in audible speech, or three times: Once audible, once whispered (yielding *whispered EMG*), once silently mouthed. The number of recording sessions per speaker varied between 1 and 32. As for the EMG-PIT corpus, the 50 BASE and SPEC utterances in each part were recorded in random order. In all experiments, the BASE sentences are used as test set, and the SPEC sentences are used for training or adaptation. Since the properties of the EMG-PIT corpus and EMG-UKA corpus are similar, we refrained from setting aside an evaluation set based on the EMG-UKA corpus. Table 3.3 displays a summary of the EMG-UKA corpus.

3.2.3 The EMG-ARRAY Data Corpus

The EMG-ARRAY corpus was recorded with the recording system described in 3.1.2. Since so far no established results on the optimal size, shape, and placement of the electrode arrays exists, we recorded a development data set com-

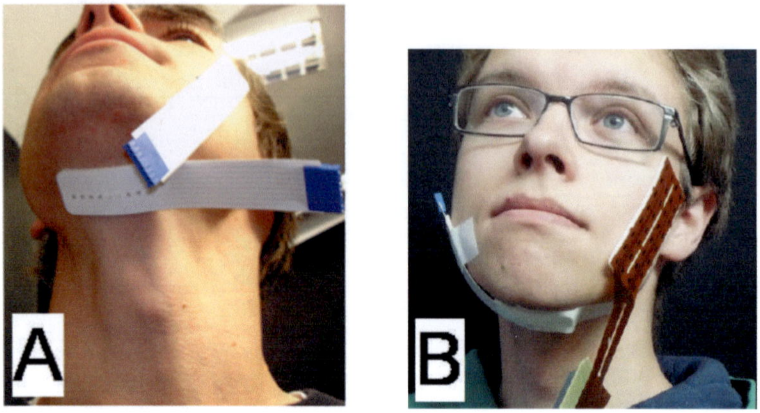

Figure 3.7 – Array placement for the 16-channel *Setup A* (left) and the 40-channel *Setup B* (right)

prising two setups, which are shown in figure 3.7: *Setup A* uses two 8-channel arrays on the chin and on the cheek, following the recording positions of the single-electrode setup as much as the shape of the arrays permits. In particular, we performed side experiments showing that the chin array, which captures signals of the tongue muscles, is necessary to achieve good recognition rates. The 16 channels resulting from this electrode setup were recorded in unipolar derivation. For *Setup B*, the cheek array is replaced with a larger array having 4×8 electrodes. The chin array remains in its place. With setup B we achieved a cleaner signal using bipolar derivation, resulting in a total of 35 channels: 7 channels come from the chin array, and $4 \cdot 7 = 28$ channels come from the cheek array.

Besides varying the array placement, a subset of sessions with an extended amount of data was recorded. For these sessions we recorded 160 training sentences, based on the original sentence lists of the EMG-PIT corpus, and 20 test sentences. In order not to increase the testing vocabulary, the 20 test sentences consist of the original BASE test sentence set repeated twice, however the 160 training sentences are unique. Each of these 180-sentence sessions contains a subset of 50 sentences which is compatible to the structure of the sessions of the EMG-PIT corpus.

This yields a development set consisting of four *non-disjoint* data subsets: The *A-1* subset consists of the 50-sentence sessions recorded with array placement A, and the *A-2* subset consists of the 180-sentence sessions recorded with array

Speaking mode	Average data length per session, in seconds Train	Test	Total	sessions / speakers
Development Set (audible EMG only)				
A-1 (50 sent.)	142	37	179	7/3
A-2 (180 sent.)	505	72	579	3/2
B-1 (50 sent.)	149	42	191	7/6
B-2 (180 sent.)	571	83	654	4/4
Total amount of data: 1:34 hours				
Evaluation Set				
B-1 (50 sent.)				
audible EMG	160	42	202	12/10
silent EMG	161	42	203	
B-2 (180 sent.)				
audible EMG	587	84	671	12/10
silent EMG	589	84	673	
Total amount of data: 4:29 hours				

Table 3.4 – EMG-ARRAY data corpus. Note that some of the 50-sentence sessions of the development set, and all 50-sentence sessions of the evaluation set, are subsets of a 180-sentence session.

placement A. Similarly, we have the *B-1* and *B-2* subsets. All recordings of the development corpus consist of audible EMG only.

During the course of the initial experiments, we showed that the B-2 setup yields better results than the other setups [WSJS13]. Therefore, we recorded an evaluation corpus of 12 sessions based on the B-2 setup, including recordings of silent speech as well: as for the other corpora, we recorded identical sentence sets for the audible and silent speaking modes. Each session contains a subset compatible to the B-1 corpus, i.e. exhibiting 40 training sentences and 10 test sentences per speaking mode. In order to avoid undue strain on the subjects, and since we did not expect any new insights, we did not include whispered speech in the EMG-ARRAY corpus.

The full EMG-ARRAY corpus is summarized in table 3.4.

Chapter 4

The Baseline EMG-based Speech Recognizer

This chapter presents and analyses the baseline system which was available at the beginning of this thesis [Jou08]; it was the first EMG-based speech recognition system ever which used phones as modeling units and could thus recognize arbitrary vocabulary. We report how the baseline system performs on our corpora, optimize several of its parameters, and present an analysis on its capabilities. For the latter purpose, we develop a recognition setup for frame-based classification of phones and phonetic features.

4.1 System Structure

The structure of the EMG-based speech recognizer is charted in figure 4.1. The EMG recognition extends the setup of a conventional speech recognizer, which is shown in figure 2.11, in particular by the use of acoustic data for bootstrapping. Also, in EMG-based speech recognition we do not train an acoustic model, but rather a ***myoelectric model***.

The four main blocks of the recognition system are: signal capturing and feature extraction, training, decoding, and the bootstrapping of the system, which is not at all very different from the acoustic case. Like conventional speech recognizers, our system integrates linguistic (language model and dictionary) information. All recognition experiments in this thesis were performed with the Janus Recognition Toolkit (JRTk) [FGH+97], using the Ibis decoder [SMFW01]. Below

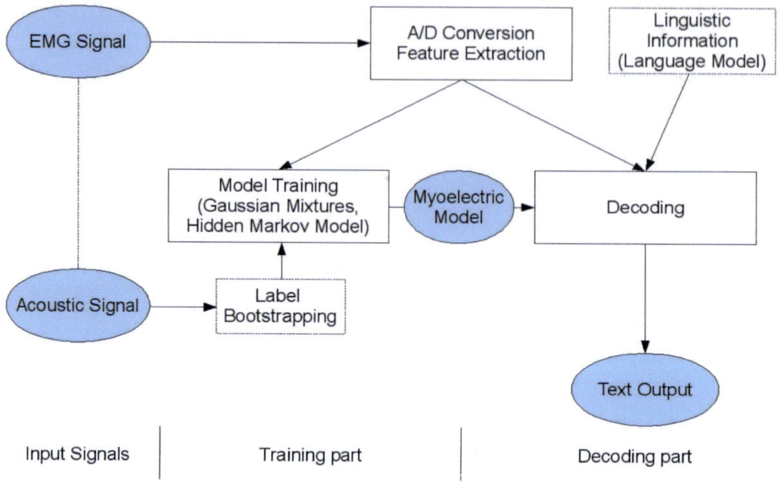

Figure 4.1 – Structure of the baseline EMG recognition system

we give a detailed description of the components of the baseline system, with the exception of the signal capturing part, which is covered in section 3.1.

4.1.1 Label Bootstrapping

The term "Label Bootstrapping" refers to the process of obtaining subphone-level time alignments ("labels") of the training data, where the term "subphone" stands for the beginning, middle, and end of a phone, see section 2.3.2. These time-alignments are required at two stages: First, we compute a Linear Discriminant Analysis transformation on the preprocessed training data, which requires information about the assignment of feature frames to the classes to be discriminated. Second, we use time-alignments for the initialization of the GMMs which form the recognizer model structure. In this chapter, we only describe the most simple case of obtaining time alignments for the audible EMG training utterances. In chapter 6 we detail the process of bootstrapping a *silent* speech EMG recognizer.

For *label bootstrapping*, we use the acoustic data which has been recorded in parallel with the EMG data, following [JSW$^+$06]. This acoustic data is forced-aligned with a standard Broadcast News (BN) speech recognizer based on the Janus Recognition Toolkit [YW00]. The recognizer uses a feature preprocessing based on Mel-Frequency Cepstral Coefficients with Vocal Tract Length Normal-

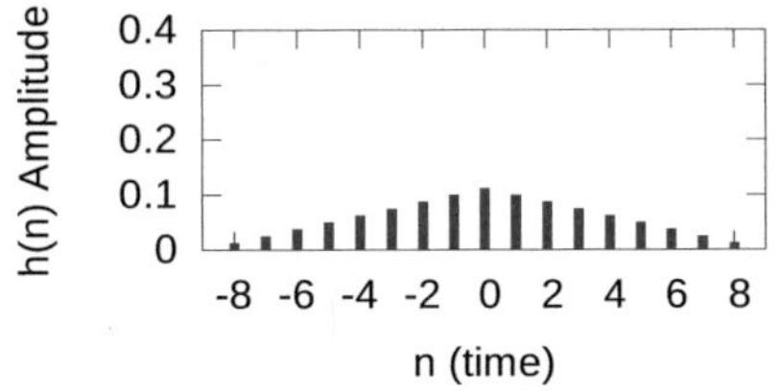

Figure 4.2 – The moving average filter which separates HF and LF components in the raw EMG signal

ization and Cepstral Mean Subtraction, after which Linear Discriminant Analysis dimensionality reduction on a 15-frames (-7 ...+7) context is performed. The acoustic model is context-dependent using two context phones per side ("quintphones"), contexts are clustered as described in section 2.3.4, yielding 6000 distributions sharing 2000 codebooks. The baseline performance of this acoustic speech recognizer is 10.2% Word Error Rate (WER) on the clean speech condition (F0) of the official BN test set [YW00, JSW+06]. The computed time-alignments from this system can be used directly to initialize the EMG models.

4.1.2 Feature Extraction

The feature extraction for the recognizer was established in [JSW+06]. It is based on *time-domain* features, which describes a very broad set of features sharing the property of being based on a time-domain representation of the signal, as opposed to features which are derived e.g. from a frequency-based or wavelet-based signal representation.

Five time-domain features per EMG channel are used, as follows. Assume that $x[n]$ is the incoming signal with normalized mean. We first filter $x[n]$ with a 17-point weighted moving average filter H, whose impulse response is charted in figure 4.2. We call the filtered EMG signal $w[n]$ the *low-frequency signal.* The remainder $p[n] := x[n] - w[n]$ is the *high-frequency signal,* its absolute (*rectified*) value is $r[n] := |p[n]|$. We point out that $w[n]$ and $p[n]$ are still time-domain signals. One can equivalently describe this filtering operation as a double application of a simple nine-point averaging filter, i.e. one obtains $w[n]$ by the following computation:

$$w[n] = \frac{1}{9} \sum_{k=-4}^{4} v[n+k], \text{ where } v[n] = \frac{1}{9} \sum_{k=-4}^{4} x[n+k]. \tag{4.1}$$

We now compute the following features: From the low-frequency signal, we compute its frame-based time-domain mean and power, and from the high-frequency signal, we compute the frame-based time-domain rectified mean, power, and zero-crossing rate. The combination of these features is called **TD0**, where "TD" stands for "time-domain", and the number 0 indicates that no context information is considered at feature level [WS10].

Now we use the following definitions from [JSW+06]: For any given input signal **y**, $\mathbf{M_y}$ is its frame-based time-domain mean, $\mathbf{P_y}$ is its frame-based power, and $\mathbf{z_y}$ is its frame-based zero-crossing rate. Now the feature **TD0** can be written as follows:

$$\mathbf{TD0} = [\mathbf{M_w}, \mathbf{P_w}, \mathbf{P_r}, \mathbf{z_p}, \mathbf{M_r}]. \tag{4.2}$$

Frame size and frame shift are set to 27 ms respectively 10 ms. The frame shift of 10ms is standard in acoustic speech recognition (see e.g. [HAH01]).

It was shown in [JSW+06] that context information is required for optimal recognition. We flexibly integrate context information by performing a stacking of adjacent feature frames with a specified context width k obtaining an enlarged feature vector: For an input sequence of features $f[n]$, we define the *stacked feature* with context k by

$$S(\mathbf{f}, k) = \tilde{f}[n], \tag{4.3}$$

where for each frame $\tilde{f}[n]$:

$$\tilde{f}[n] = [f[n-k], f[n-k+1], \ldots, f[n], \ldots, f[n+k]].$$

This means that our five-dimensional input feature is extended to $5 \cdot (2k+1)$ dimensions. We fix the value k at 10 and obtain the channel-wise feature **TD10** $=$ $S(\mathbf{TD0}, 10)$. Since the channel-wise features are now also stacked, we end up with $5 \cdot 5 \cdot 21 = 525$ dimensions in the **TD10** feature. Note that different context widths are used in the experiments based on the EMG-ARRAY corpus described in chapter 7.

Finally a linear discriminant analysis (LDA) transformation is computed. For this step we require a time-alignment of the training utterances, assigning one sub-phone class to each frame. Since our English dictionary uses 45 phones, we have $3 \cdot 45 + 1 = 136$ phone classes including the silence class. When the LDA transformation is computed, we retain the 12 most discriminant dimensions.

We note at this point that many of the above parameters may be varied, causing changes in the recognizer performance. For the initial experiments reported in this chapter, we chose our parameters so that they give optimal results on the development corpora, see section 4.3 for more information about the optimization of parameters.

4.1.3 Modeling and Training

The baseline recognizer uses three-state left-to-right Hidden Markov Models (HMMs), where each state represents a context-independent subphone (see section 2.3.2). These HMMs thus follow the setup set out in section 2.3.2, see figure 2.12. The emission probabilities of the HMM states are Gaussian Mixture Models (GMMs), transition probabilities are not trained.

The training of the recognizer consists of two steps:

- First, we initialize the Gaussian Mixture Models (GMMs) which underly the HMM states. This is done by merge-and-split training [UNGH00].
- Second, we perform four iterations of Viterbi training.

The merge-and-split initialization step uses time-alignments which are computed from the parallel acoustic data as long as audible EMG is concerned, see section 4.1.1 for more details. During Viterbi training, improved time-alignments are computed from the EMG data as part of the Baum-Welch optimization rules (see section 2.3.5). Finally, the output of the training step is a set of Gaussian mixture models, one for each subphone which occurs in the training data.

4.1.4 Language Modeling and Decoding

For decoding, we apply a standard trigram language model trained on Broadcast News data. On the test set, the trigram perplexity of the language model is 24.24. The decoding uses time-synchronous Viterbi beam search, as described in section 2.3.6. After a first hypothesis is generated, optional lattice rescoring based on a matrix of word penalty and language model weighting parameters can be performed in order to obtain optimal recognition results; in this thesis, lattice rescoring is *not* used. Evaluation of the baseline system is performed on the single-electrode corpora (i.e. EMG-PIT and EMG-UKA). As described in section 3.2, we always use the batch of speaker-specific audible SPEC utterances as training set, and the audible BASE utterances as testing set.

We follow [JSW+06] in limiting the decoding vocabulary to the 108 words appearing in the test set. The limited decoding vocabulary is a consequence of the small amount of session-dependent training data provided by the EMG-PIT and EMG-UKA corpora, the (newer) EMG-ARRAY corpus contains a set of larger sessions. Also, in chapter 8, results on *session-independent* systems are presented, where we have the opportunity to work with a much larger amount of training data than in the session-dependent case, and where the decoding vocabulary is

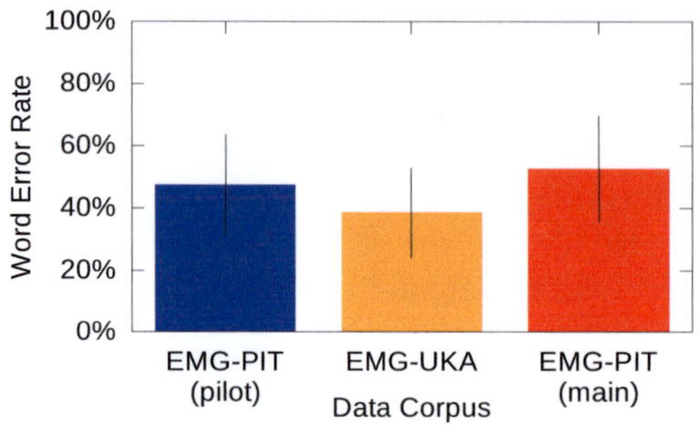

Figure 4.3 – Overview of Word Error Rates with the baseline system. Bars indicate standard deviation, computed over all sessions.

consequently enlarged to 2102 words—the full set of words in the EMG-PIT and EMG-UKA corpora.

4.2 Baseline Results

We begin the evaluation of our baseline system with an overview of the recognition performance on the audible part of the EMG-PIT corpus and the single-session part of the EMG-UKA corpus. All experiments are *session-dependent*, which means that training and testing is performed on the same session. We compute results on all single-electrode corpora, including the evaluation corpus, to serve as a reference for later chapters.

As performance measure we use the *Word Error Rate* (WER), which is given by aligning the hypothesis and the reference text at word level and then counting the numbers N_I, N_D, N_S of insertions, deletions, and substitutions: thus we compute the *Levenshtein distance* between hypothesis and reference. The WER is then defined as

$$\mathrm{WER} = \frac{N_I + N_D + N_S}{N} \cdot 100\%, \tag{4.4}$$

where N is the total number of words in the reference. A smaller WER means that the recognition accuracy improves. Clearly, this measure is only applicable if the reference text is known, which is the case for all our corpora. The WER for one session is always averaged over all testing utterances of that session.

The average WER of the recognizer on the three corpora is given in figure 4.3 and table 4.1. For this experiment we chose optimal settings, where optimization was performed on the development corpora only, see section 4.3 for details.

Corpus	Number of sessions	Average Word Error Rate	Standard Deviation
EMG-UKA	61	38.6%	± 17.0%
EMG-PIT (pilot)	28	47.5%	± 16.2%
EMG-PIT (main)	62	52.6%	± 14.3%

Table 4.1 – Word Error Rates and standard deviations of the baseline system for the three single-electrode corpora

As a general observation, we see that the WER on the EMG-UKA corpus is lower than on the two parts of the EMG-PIT corpus. Indeed we made the observation that the analog high-pass filter of the amplifier which we used for the EMG-UKA corpus seems to perform better in removing low-frequency movement artifacts. However, the result should not be considered significant, since the sets of speakers for the two corpora have substantially different characteristics (see section 3.2): The EMG-PIT corpus contains one or two sessions per speaker, and the speakers had no prior experience in silent speech. In the EMG-UKA corpus, we have up to 32 sessions for one experienced speaker, but there are also speakers who recorded just one session.

In figure 4.4 we see a breakdown of the results on the EMG-PIT pilot corpus and on the EMG-UKA corpus; for the former, we have the results by session, on the latter, we average over all sessions of the respective speakers and give the standard deviation where more than one session was used. It can be observed that the results by speaker vary greatly, for example, on the EMG-PIT corpus the best session WER is 20%, and the worst session WER is 78%. However, most speakers achieve rather consistent results across all their recorded sessions, with the notable exception of speaker 7 from the EMG-UKA corpus. So far we cannot answer the question what makes a speaker a good speaker: One may assume the influence of skin conditions and muscle properties, as well as articulation idiosyncrasies.

4.3 Parameter Optimization

As machine learning systems are wont to do, the EMG-based speech recognizer has a large number of parameters which may be chosen within a wide numerical range. This section deals with the influence of parameter variations on the recognition results. The purpose of this section is notably *not* to optimize every single parameter of the system, which we believe to be pointless at the current stage of development of the system. We rather intend to show that parameter variations

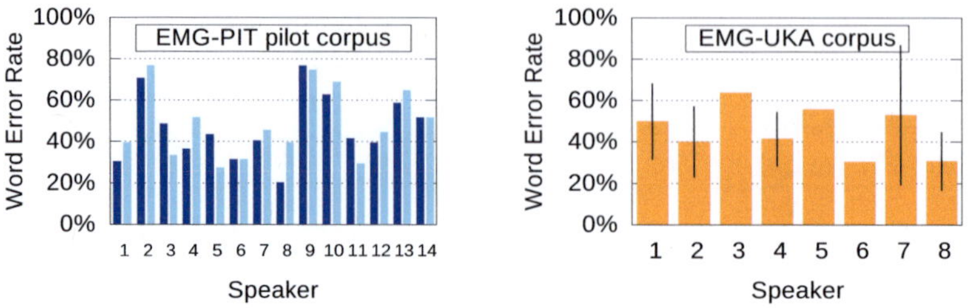

Figure 4.4 – Overview of Word Error Rates by Speaker for the Development Corpora. Results on the EMG-PIT pilot corpus are given by session, on the EMG-UKA corpus, we averaged over all sessions of each speaker. Bars indicate standard deviation.

yield "continuous" changes in the Word Error Rate, thus a rough optimization of the most important parameters should be sufficient in order to guarantee robust results. In particular, for many minor parameters, the system behaves robustly when these parameters are (moderately) perturbed. We take these observations as an indicator of the stability of our setup and for the validity of our experiments. All experiments are performed on the pilot part of the EMG-PIT corpus and on the Single-Session part of the EMG-UKA corpus.

We identified the following major parameters in the system:

- The time-domain feature preprocessing (**TD0**)
- Context width during the creation of the **TD**n feature
- Number of retained dimensions after LDA
- Merge-and-split parameters (e.g. the threshold amount of training data beyond which a Gaussian can be split)
- Number of iterations during Viterbi training.

The greatest parameter variation can be performed in the feature extraction part, on which we focus in this section. We also varied the set of parameters during training (i.e. the merge-and-split parameters and the Viterbi training settings, including the beam settings and the number of iterations). Here we found that as long as the parameters remain within a certain range, no clear optimum is observed, eventually we decided to keep the standard settings unchanged.

EMG feature preprocessing in the context of speech recognition was already researched before work on this thesis started. Jou et al. showed that time-domain features of the kind presented above are superior to a collection of frequency-based features, in particular when context information is used

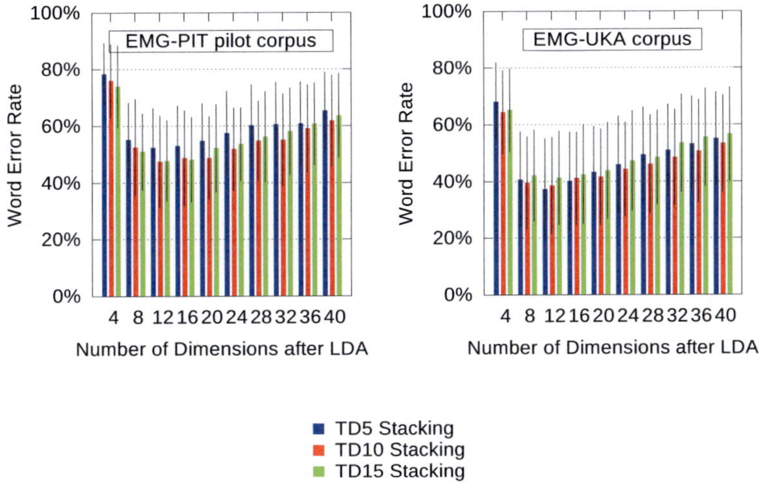

Figure 4.5 – Average Word Error Rates for the development corpora, for different numbers of retained dimensions after LDA. Bars indicate standard deviation.

[JSW+06]. Clearly, there are many variants and extensions of the above time-domain features, and it exceeds the scope of this thesis to investigate them all. Notwithstanding, we ran several experiments with some variations of these features, without observing significant changes in the performance of the recognizer, among these feature variations were inclusion of features like the waveform length [HLW03] or different moving average filters. We assume that as long as one limits oneself to the kind of frame-based time-domain features which we present here, there is a wide range of features which yield similar average performance. If it is desired to improve beyond this level, one should consider more advanced signal processing methods, which we do in chapter 7.

The parameters which we found to yield substantial WER changes are the feature dimensionality after LDA application and the **TD** stacking width. Figure 4.5 shows the WER for different numbers of retained dimensions after LDA, and for three **TD** stacking widths (5, 10, and 15). We consistently observe a minimum WER at the dimensionality 12.

The feature space dimensionality impacts the training performance due to the "Curse of Dimensionality", explained in section 2.3.1: When the model dimensionality is high and the amount of training data is fixed, increasing the dimensionality of the feature space will cause a reduction of recognition accuracy (i.e. an increasing WER). Indeed this is observed from figure 4.5: When using more

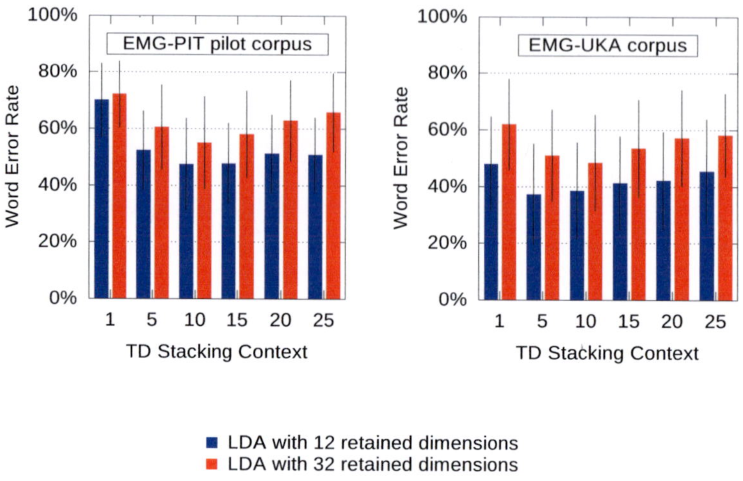

Figure 4.6 – Average Word Error Rates for the development corpora, for different context stacking widths. Bars indicate standard deviation.

than 12 dimensions after LDA, the WER rises, independently of the stacking width. So we conclude that for the given amount of training data, the optimal feature space size is indeed 12, no matter whether we add extra information. This result is rather consistent across speakers and sessions. We will reinvestigate this problem in light of our high-dimensional *EMG arrays* in chapter 7.

Finally, we investigate a related factor, namely the optimal context stacking width. Figure 4.6 shows the resulting word error rates for 12 and 32 retained dimensions after LDA application and for stacking widths ranging from 1 to 25 (note that we do not use **TD0** features, i.e. no stacking at all, since this would result in only 25 dimensions prior to LDA, which we cannot sensibly project to a 32-dimensional subspace; however it is clear from figure 4.6 that using no context stacking would yield suboptimal results anyway). We observe that for 32 dimensions, the optimal stacking width is 10. For 12 dimensions, the result is less clear: For the EMG-PIT pilot corpus, the optimal stacking width is again 10, for the EMG-UKA corpus, the optimum is at 5, which gives poorer results on the EMG-PIT corpus. We observe the tendency that the optimum stacking context width is around 10, so as a compromise, we use **TD10** as final feature for our further experiments.

4.4 Phone-Level Analysis

The system we presented in section 4.1 is composed of several components, as charted in figure 4.1. Consequently, the results from sections 4.2 and 4.3 are based on a fusion of "knowledge" from these components: In particular, the vocabulary size is rather small compared to large-scale conventional speech recognition, so the vocabulary and the language model add a great amount of information to the EMG features.

In this section we report on the recognizer performance at the *phone* level [WS11a]. This means that we forgo our HMM modeling, as well as the language model, and perform a purely frame-based recognition of phones. With this experiment we intend to gain a deeper understanding of the properties and capabilites of our unit modeling, particularly when compared with standard acoustic speech recognition. Additionally, the results will guide us on our way towards improving the recognizer with a versatile modeling method, as presented in chapter 5.

The detailed technical specifications of the frame-based phone recognizer are as follows: Our feature preprocessing remains as described in section 4.1.2, using **TD10** features and LDA for dimensionality reduction to 12 retained dimensions. We create session-dependent Gaussian Mixture Models (GMMs) for each of our 45 phones[1]. The GMMs are initialized with merge-and-split training based on the acoustic time-alignments, followed by four iterations of the EM algorithm for GMMs [Bis07, Chapter 9]. These GMMs therefore correspond to the *unit models* of the full recognition system. During training we do *not* alter the assignment of signal frames to phones, i.e. new Viterbi alignments are not computed; instead, the acoustic phone-level alignments computed in section 4.1.1 are taken as ground truth both for the training and testing phase. Testing consists of matching the hypothesis of the GMM classifier against the frame-level reference taken from the alignment. Note that we remove all silence frames from the training and testing data in order to avoid unbalanced results: Since speakers frequently made a short pause between pressing the recording button and actually starting to speak, the "Silence" phone is by far the most frequent phone of both corpora, and it is very easy to be distinguished from non-silence phones.

On the pilot part of the EMG-PIT corpus, we achieve a phone accuracy of 16.8%, on the EMG-UKA corpus, the accuracy is 16.6%. Of course, despite the removal of silence frames, these results are based on a highly unbalanced class distribution:

[1]We also created subphone models, i.e. models for the beginning, middle, and end parts of a phone. In this case we observed that the parts of a phone are often confused, across phones, the confusion patterns are very similar to the phone model case.

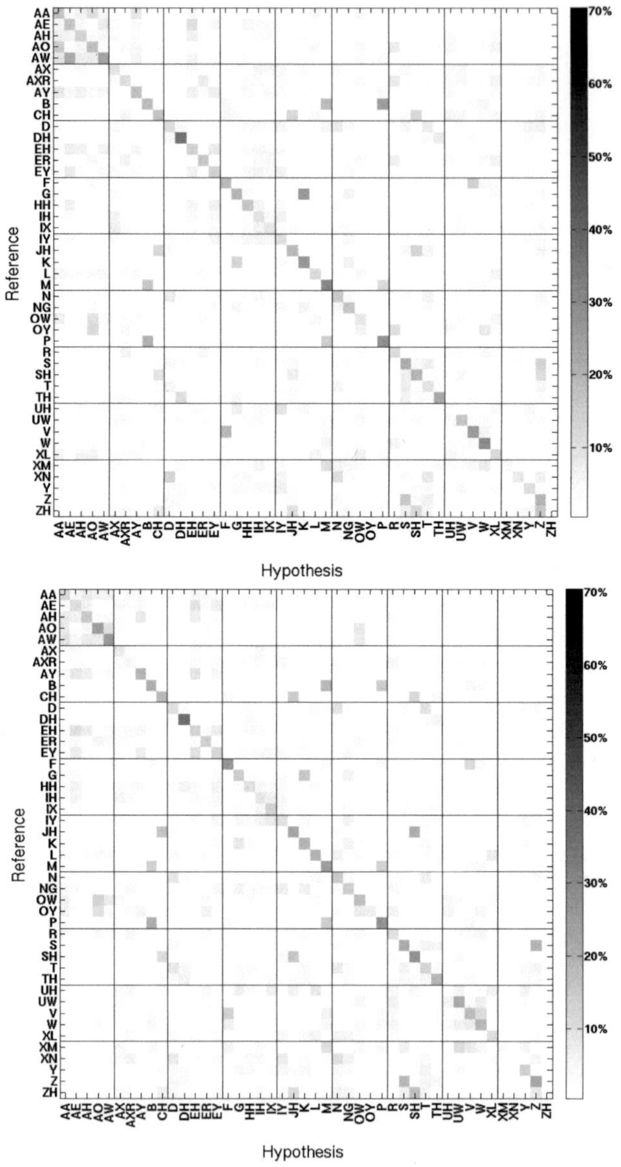

Figure 4.7 – Confusion matrices for frame-based phone recognition based on EMG data: EMG-PIT Corpus, pilot part (top), EMG-UKA corpus (bottom)

The number of frames per class in the training data ranges from 100 to 6500 on the pilot part of the EMG-PIT corpus, and from 250 to 15000 on the (larger) EMG-UKA corpus. Still, we are able to draw conclusions based on the *phone-level confusion*, i.e. we consider the distribution of recognition errors across different phones.

The phone-level confusion is graphically represented in figure 4.7. Each row represents a reference phone, and each column represents a hypothesized phone. The darkness of a cell indicates the frequency of this confusion: In a perfect system, all cells on the diagonal would be black, and all other cells would be white. All plotted confusions are *relative*, in the sense that the rows of the confusion matrix sum to one.

We observe that vowels are quite frequently confused with each other, the most obvious case is the set of "A-like" vowels in the upper left, including [AA] (as in *far*), [AE] (as is *bat*), [AO] (as in *flaw*), [AH] (as in *fun*), and even the diphthong [AW] (as in *power*). Note that a certain amount of confusion is unavoidable particularly when diphthongs are concerned, since their realization inevitably stretches over more than one frame. Additionally, it must be assumed that the acoustic alignments representing the ground truth are not always perfect: some phones might have been mispronounced by the speakers, the articulation boundaries between certain vowels might vary depending on the accent of the speaker, and HMMs are known for issues in boundary frame assignment.

We now consider consonants. We observe several major "confusion groups", which we define as groups of phones which are frequently mutually confused. The bilabial consonants [B], [P], and [M] fall into one confusion group: On the EMG-UKA corpus, of all [B]s, around 22% are recognized as [B], 20.9% are recognized as [M], and 16.4% are recognized as [P]. A similar pattern holds for [P]s and [M]s.

The alveolar consonants [D], [N], and [T] form a very similar group, for example, of all [D]s, 11% are recognized as [D], 9.7% are confused with [N], and another 9.3% are confused with [T]. Further confusion groups include [G] and [K], [S] and [Z], which are the voiceless and voiced alveolar fricative, respectively, and [CH], [JH], and [SH] (as in *church, John, shell*).

From the confusion groups, we draw the conclusion that the *place* of articulation is detected relatively well, but that detecting *voicing* or the *manner* of articulation (e.g. plosive versus nasal) are problematic. This can be explained by considering how different phones are articulated, as detailed in section 2.2.2: The place of articulation is determined by the large-scale movement of the articulators, so it should be well-detectable from the activity of the articulatory muscles.

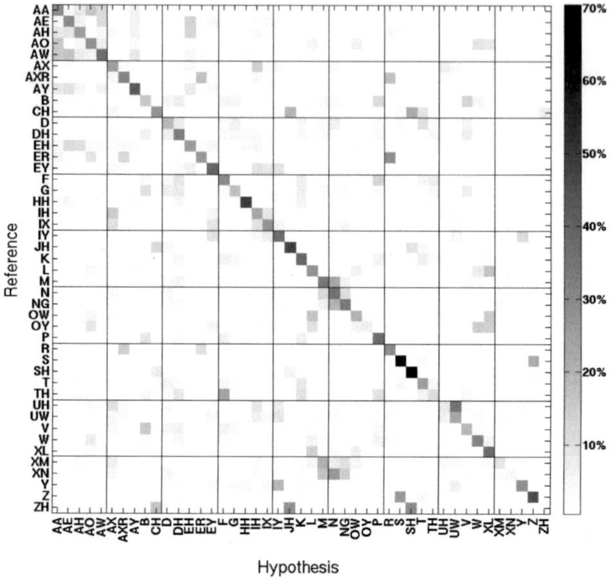

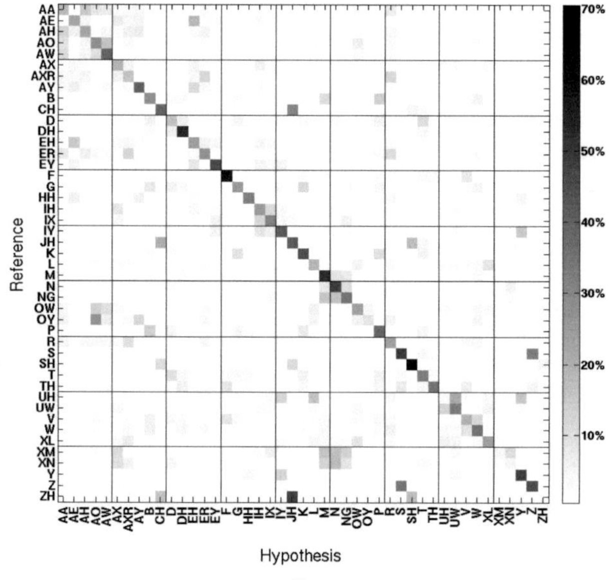

Figure 4.8 – Confusion matrices for frame-based phone recognition based on *acoustic* data: EMG-PIT Corpus, pilot part (top), EMG-UKA corpus (bottom)

Category	EMG data		Acoustic data	
	EMG-PIT (pil.)	EMG-UKA	EMG-PIT (pil.)	EMG-UKA
Manner	47.73%	47.65%	69.38%	75.92%
Position	55.59%	51.24%	56.48%	66.43%
Voicing	62.63%	63.37%	80.77%	80.14%

Table 4.2 – Classification accuracies for phonetic feature classes on EMG data and acoustic data.

The manner of articulation obviously also depends on the configuration of the articulators, but here the differences are more subtle (compare for example the sounds [b] and [m]). One furthermore notes from this example that in some articulatory movements are partially shared between phones, in the case of [b] and [m], the initial part of these phones requires *identical* articulatory movements, namely closing the lips. This would cause high confusion between some of the frames belonging to the phones [b] and [m].

Finally, voicing depends on glottal activity, which is not captured by our EMG setup and it therefore very hard to recognize. Yet, the result that in whispered speech, minimal pairs differing only in the phonological voicing of a single phone can be discerned (see section 2.2.3), gives hope that there are also differences in the articulation of voiced and voiceless consonants which are recognizable from the EMG signal, even in silent speech. This expectation is supported by current results with the PMA technology [HBC$^+$13].

The EMG phone confusion patterns reported here differ substantially from those observed in acoustic speech recognition, where one typically observes that voicing and manner of articulation are recognized very well, but that confusion is possible among low-energy sounds like [P], [T], and [K] [Kir99, Chapter 3.2.2], which is not so much the case for EMG since these sounds require very different articulator configuations. For comparison, figure 4.8 shows confusion results on the acoustic data of the EMG-PIT (pilot) and EMG-UKA corpus, which supports this observation and also shows an additional confusion group consisting of the nasals [M], [N], and [NG], which is not present for EMG. The accuracy of the acoustics-based system is much higher, at 33.0% and 35.5% for the EMG-PIT and EMG-UKA corpus, respectively.

To complete the study on frame-based recognition, frame-based classification of *phonetic features* instead of phones is performed: this means that phones are grouped into classes based on certain phonetic categories. In the next chapter an exact definition of phonetic features is given, for now, it suffices to say that we are interested in the broad distinctions discussed above: voicing, manner, and position of articulation. The phonetic categories are defined as follows: For voicing, there are two obvious classes (*voiced* and *unvoiced*), where all vowels fall into the *voiced* category. For the manner of articulation, we take the following categories from the IPA chart (see section 2.2.2): *plosive, nasal, fricative, affricate, approximant.* The articulation positions which are to be distinguished are: *bilabial, labiodental, alveolar, palatal, velar, glottal.* These classes follow the pattern set by the underlying EMG-based speech recognizer taken from [Jou08], they do not fully cover the entire IPA chart since some articulations (e.g. pharyngeal and uvular) do not occur in English language, and some others are only covered by a single phone (for example, the only lateral approximant would be [l], so we adjoin it to the group of approximants).

The results are summarized in table 4.2. Since the sample sizes by class vary, we average the accuracies over the classes: For *each class*, we compute the ratio of correctly classified frames to the total number of frames which the acoustic reference alignment assigns to this class, and then compute the average of these accuracies. This means that in all cases, the chance level for classification is $\frac{1}{\text{\# classes}}$. Confusion plots are shown in figure 4.9.

The observations from the phone-based system are confirmed: On the EMG-PIT corpus, the articulation position is recognized from EMG data with 55.59% average accuracy, and the manner of articulation is recognized with only 47.73% average accuracy, despite the fact that there are six position classes and only five manner classes. Voicing is rather hard to recognize, with only 62.63% accuracy on two classes. Yet, this is above chance level. The results are similar on both corpora, but differ very much from the results on acoustic data, where the manner of articulation is much better recognized than the position of articulation, and voicing is recognized best of all.

Finally, the PF confusion plots in figure 4.9 reveal a notable pattern. For EMG-based classification of the articulation position, there are two visible confusion groups: Bilabial and labiodental consonants are frequently confused, and so are consonants assigned to one of the other four articulation positions. Confusions *between* the groups are less frequent. We derive from section 2.2.2 that these two groups differ in the activity of the lips, which are obviously central for articulation of bilabial and labiodental consonants, but are less active in the other cases, where the tongue plays a more central role.

For the classification of manner of articulation, and for the acoustic case, no clear plattern is observed, and the single-electrode setup clearly does not suffice to determine which muscles cause the confusion and recognition patterns we observe. Yet, it is clear that EMG-based phone classification recognizes articulatory move-

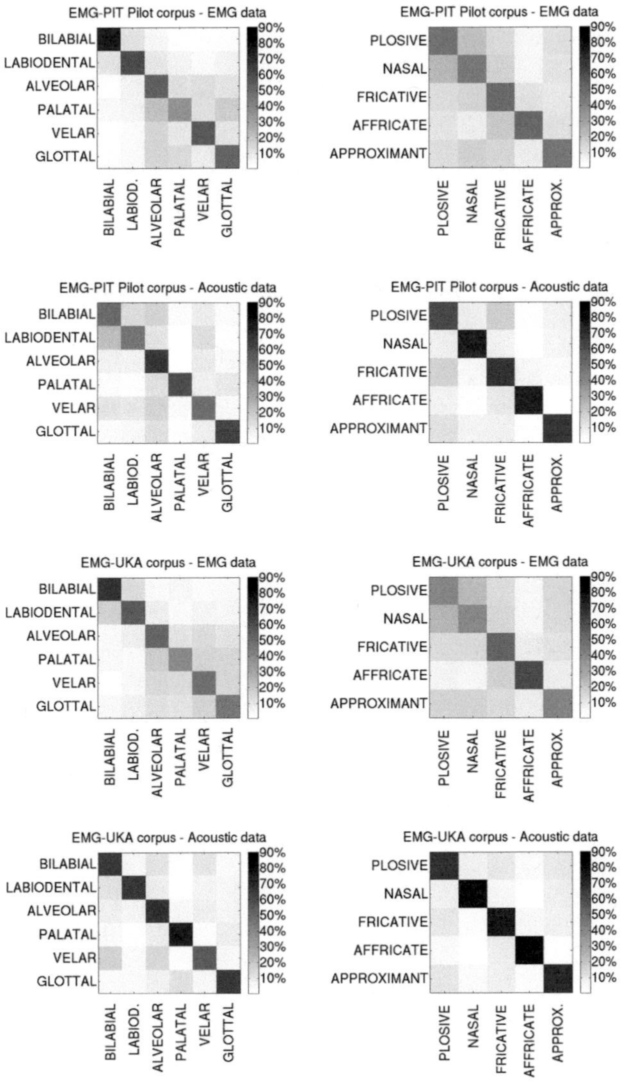

Figure 4.9 – Confusion plots for phonetic feature recognition. The plots show the confusion for *position* resp. *manner* of articulation, on both corpora and for EMG signals and acoustic signals.

ments in a consistent manner: Even though the accuracy is substantially lower than for acoustics, this is an encouraging result, since it proves that our stated goal of eventually extracting and classifying articulatory movements is realistic.

Chapter 5

Phonetic Features and the Feature Bundling Algorithm

In this chapter we introduce a new and innovative modeling structure for the EMG-based speech recognizer. The new models are based on the fusion of multiple knowledge sources in form of Phonetic Feature models, which represent partial information about phones. The key novelty is that dependencies between phonetic features are modeled, yielding ***Bundled Phonetic Features*** *(BDPF), which reduce the Word Error Rate of our recognizer by up to 40.8% relative.*

5.1 Phonetic Features as Modeling Units

The EMG-based speech recognizer which was presented in chapter 4 is based on *context-independent subphones* as modeling units. This means that each frame of the EMG signal is regarded as the realization of the beginning, middle, or end state of a phone. In order to improve results, a new modeling paradigm is developed, which is presented in this chapter. It is based upon three principles:

- **Phonetic Feature modeling** As demonstrated in chapter 4, *phonetic features* (PFs) can serve as classes to be discriminated by a frame-based recognizer. Any phone can be described as a set of phonetic features (compare section 2.2.2), so it should be possible to combine the results of PF classifiers for phone classification and, consequently, for continuous speech recognition. Prior results, reviewed in section 5.1.1, show that this concept can yield better results than standard phone-based modeling.

«HELLO WORLD» → Pronunciation Dictionary Lookup

Phones	h	e	l	ou	w	er	l	d
⇩ Phonetic Features ⇩								
Alveolar			✓				✓	✓
Glottal	✓							
Plosive								✓
Fricative	✓							
Approximant			✓		✓		✓	
...								
Vowel		✓		✓		✓		
Front (Vowel)		✓						
Round (Vowel)				✓				

Figure 5.1 – Derivation of Phonetic Features from phones

- **Data-driven model optimization** We wish to create optimized models which capture the articulatory variability of the data *and* may be properly trained with a relatively small amount of training samples. Context-dependent modeling (compare section 2.3.4) is the standard answer to this question as far as acoustic speech recognition is concerned, however the limited training data amount precludes its application at least in our session-dependent systems.
- **Data reuse** The current EMG data corpus is relatively small compared to corpora used in classical acoustic speech recognition. Therefore it is greatly desirable to find a way to make efficient use of training data by *reusing* it in different contexts.

In this chapter, these principles are combined to form a new and innovative modeling structure for our recognizer, which we first presented in [SW10]. It is shown that compared to the baseline system presented in chapter 4, this new structure yields a relative WER improvement of up to 40.8% relative.

5.1.1 A Review on Phonetic Features

As in section 4.4, we define *Phonetic Features (PFs)* as properties of phones, like the place or the manner of articulation. This assignment is canonic, it is derived directly from the standard IPA charts for vowels (figure 2.7) and consonants (figure 2.8).

Phonetic Features have been studied for many decades, albeit under different names. The original theory of *distinctive features* is primarily attributed to the Russian-American linguist Roman O. Jakobson [Wil66], who developed his framework more than 50 years ago ([JFH52], cited according to [HOW06]). The goal of this distinctive features theory was, of course, not computer-based speech recognition, but rather understanding the properties of language: for example, it was asked how differences between words are perceived by a listener. Classically, it is assumed that word differences are formed by contrasts between whole sounds of a word (i.e. *phonemes*, see section 2.2.2), but it might be possible that such meaning differences are conveyed by smaller contrasts, like the contrast in a single binary-valued phonetic feature, for example, by the voicing contrast in the words *bill* versus *pill* [HOW06].

In terms of computer-based speech recogntion, phonetic features were studied on a large scale by K. Kirchhoff in her doctoral dissertation [Kir99], although there exist prior studies, see [Kir99, Chapter 2.4]. In Kirchhoff's work, the term *Articulatory Features* is used, with the restricting remark: "The articulatory features we are concerned with in this thesis are not detailed numerical descriptions of the movements of articulators during speech production. Rather, they are abstract classes which characterize the most essential aspects of articulation in a highly quantized, canonical form [...]" [Kir99, Chapter 1].

Modeling the movement of the articulators may not be necessary in acoustic speech recognition, but on the long run this will certainly be a topic in EMG-based speech recognition, as it is with other modalities, for example EMA [Ric09]. Hence in order to use clear terminology, we avoid the term "articulatory features" and talk about "phonetic features" instead. This also allows to use a somewhat more general definition than Kirchhoff, where phonetic features are required to "have well-defined correlates in articulatory space" [Kir99, Chapter 2.4.2], and include purely functional phonetic features without a clear representation in articulatory space, like "Consonant" or "Syllabic".

Kirchhoff studied conventional acoustic speech recognition. PFs are understood as multi-valued variables describing properties of phone articulation. Typical PF include *Voicing*, *Manner* of articulation, *Place* of articulation, *Vowel Position* (front – back), and lip *Rounding*. The central achievements of Kirchhoff's study are an increased robustness of a hybrid phone/PF classifier compared to a standard phone-based recognizer in the presence of ambient noise, and the proof that PF models encode information which is not available in a standard phone-based recognizer. However, it is also observed that the PFs can enhance, but not replace, the original phone-based system due to "the poorer separability of phonetic classes in articulatory feature space compared to the acoustic feature space" [Kir99, Chapter 4.7]. Finally, it is hypothesized that including interdependencies between phonetic features could make the classification more robust [Kir99, Chapter 5.2].

The basic structure and implementation of the PF recognition system employed in this thesis is taken from the experiments of F. Metze [MW02, Met05], wherein the phonetic features are integrated into a conventional (acoustic, phone-based) speech recognizer by means of a *Multi-Stream* architecture. This architecture is described in detail in the following section 5.1.2. Just as Kirchhoff, Metze derives PFs from the underlying phones; in contrast to Kirchhoff, he uses *binary* PFs, e.g. the feature "Plosive" may be present (in English, this is true for the sounds [p], [b], [t], [d], [k], and [g]) or absent (this includes not only the majority of consonants, but also all vowel sounds). The derivation of binary-valued PFs from phones is displayed in figure 5.1.

Metze achieves results similar to Kirchhoff, in particular, an improved robustness towards spontaneous and hyper-articulated speech. Furthermore, discriminative training methods (e.g. *Minimum Classification Error (MCE)* [JCL97] or *Maximum Mutual Information Estimation (MMIE)*) are investigated at the PF level. As in Kirchhoff's works, it is observed that PFs cannot fully replace the original phone-based system.

This multi-stream system was first applied to EMG-based speech recognition by Szu-Chen Jou [JSW07, Jou08] as part of his PhD thesis. In [JSW07], applying the optimal PF multi-stream setup to EMG-based speech recognition is reported to yield a WER improvement of 11.8% relative, based on a single recording session of one single speaker, with 380 training sentences. In [Jou08, Chapter 4.7.8], the system is reapplied to a larger corpus, still yielding 6.2% relative improvement.

Within the context of this thesis, the main result so far is that it is worthwhile to study phonetic features not only as an analysis tool, as was done in section 4.4, but also as a modeling tool, thus realizing the first principle defined above, i.e. Phonetic Feature modeling. The first benefit which should be expected is that PF models might be better estimated when few training data is available, since the available amount of training data is divided among a smaller amount of classes. Note that for this purpose, it might not be required to form classes based on phonetic categories: it is expected that other phone groupings would also work, as long as the contained phones share some common properties which allow modeling the class as a whole. Yet, the results on PF classification from section 4.4 suggest that using phonetic features as a starting point automatically yields classes which share common properties, in both the EMG and the acoustic case. In section 5.2, we leverage these robustly estimated PF models to obtain a realization of the second principle defined above, i.e. model optimization. The

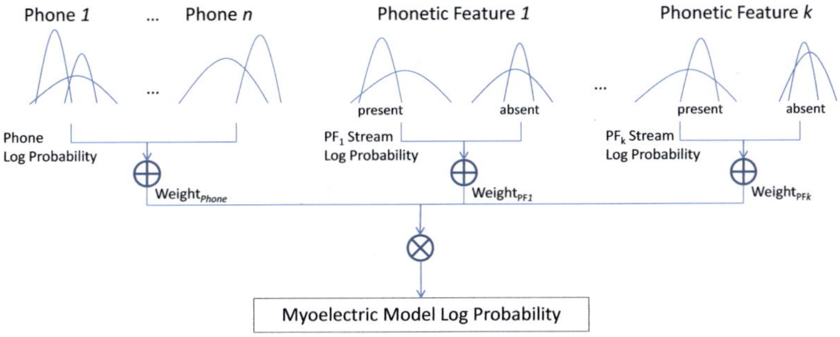

Figure 5.2 – Composition of phone scores from Phonetic Feature scores: the *multi-stream* model

question whether Phonetic Features might be more robust towards artifacts than standard phone models is beyond the scope of this study.

The remainder of this chapter is structured as follows: In section 5.1.2 we first describe and evaluate the original multi-stream PF system, which corresponds to the one applied in [Jou08]. In section 5.2, *Bundled Phonetic Feature* modeling is introduced as a key result of this study, and a detailed evaluation is performed. Finally, in section 5.3, the results are summarized and a conclusion is drawn. All experiments are session-dependent, and as in the last chapter, we use the pilot part of the EMG-PIT corpus and the EMG-UKA corpus as development data and the main part of the EMG-PIT corpus for evaluation.

5.1.2 The Multi-Stream Architecture

The structure of the *multi-stream* system originating from [Met05, Jou08] is depicted in figure 5.2. Here, the emission log probability of a phone within the HMM framework is computed as a weighted sum of log probabilities from various *streams*, i.e. knowledge sources. One knowledge source corresponds to the standard phone model, so we have a set of Gaussian Mixture Models (GMMs) corresponding to the set of phones. The other knowledge sources correspond to phonetic features, where we have the "present" and "absent" models.

Note that the following minor points are not shown in the figure: For the "Silent" phone a separate model is used, so that the silent phone affects neither the "present" nor the "absent" model of any PF, and we have models corresponding not to phones, but to subphones, i.e. the beginning, middle, or end of a phone, see section 2.3.2. This transfers to the PF modeling: Each PF stream has seven

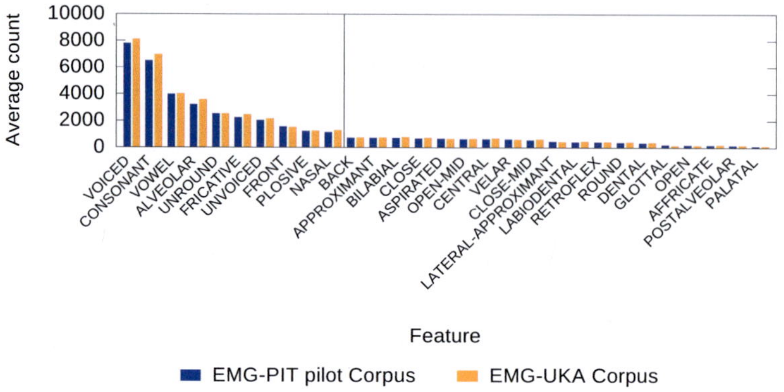

Figure 5.3 – Average number of frames per phonetic feature in the training data. The first 10 features each have more than 1,000 frames.

models for the beginning, middle, or end of a present or absent feature, plus one silence model.

As an example, the end of "H" in the word "hello" would be modeled using

- the model "H-e" (end of phone "H") in the phone stream,
- the model "Non-Alveolar-e" in the "Alveolar" stream,
- the model "Glottal-e" in the "Glottal" stream,
- the model "Non-Plosive-e" in the "Plosive" stream,
- etc.

The final score, i.e. the (negative) log-likelihood

$$-\log \mathrm{p}(x|\text{model H-e}) =: \text{Score(model H-e)},$$

of an observation x for the model "H-e" is then computed by the formula

$$\begin{aligned}\text{Score(model H-e)} = &\ \text{Weight}_{\text{Phone}} \cdot \text{Score(phone H-e)} \\ &+ \text{Weight}_{\text{Alveolar}} \cdot \text{Score(Non-Alveolar-e)} \\ &+ \text{Weight}_{\text{Glottal}} \cdot \text{Score(Glottal-e)} \\ &+ \text{Weight}_{\text{Plosive}} \cdot \text{Score(Non-Plosive-e)} \\ &+ \text{further PF scores.}\end{aligned}$$

In particular, there is *one* final score for the model "H-e", as in a conventional model. This allows a direct integration of the multi-stream architecture into the standard HMM framework for speech recognition (see section 4.1).

For the following experiments, we have to make an informed choice which phonetic features should be used for modeling. In [JSW07], eight PF streams are used in the multi-stream decoding setup. The WER improves when more streams are added, but only up to five streams, where a saturation effect is observed. This might be due to the varying amount of frames per *present* phonetic feature: only those features where sufficient training data is available are well modeled.

We counted the number of frames available for each phonetic feature per session. The average over all sessions is depicted in figure 5.3; there are ten PFs where the average number of frames exceeds 1000, with a notable leap to the eleventh PF. Out of these 10 features, two are redundant in the sense that they are exact complements of previous features: "Vowel" and "Unvoiced".

In the following experiments, the 10 most frequent PFs are used. We note that these 10 PFs do *not* fully cover all possible English articulations, for example, many articulation position from the IPA chart (see section 2.2.2) are disregarded. Since for now we just intend to use PF modeling to augment phone modeling, this is not considered a problem, we rather prefer to make sure that our models are well trained.

Since presence and absence of PFs are equally modeled in the multi-stream model, the two redundant features "Vowel" and "Unvoiced" can be left out; they are already covered by the absent complementary PFs, i.e. "Non-Consonant" and "Non-Voiced". So we obtain *eight* PF streams, the phone stream contributes as well. We make the further constraint that all PF streams must have the same weight. It is possible to learn such weights (Discriminative Model Combination [Bey00]), and experiments in acoustic speech recognition on a setup similar to our own are presented in [Met05, Chapter 7.2]. We refrain from applying Discriminative Model Combination on the PF setup developed so far since the system is substantially changed in section 5.2, where phonetic feature bundling is introduced. See section 5.2.3 for remarks on optimal stream weighting for Bundled Phonetic Features, and on the exchangability of streams.

5.1.3 Results and Analysis

We evaluate PF-based modeling on the EMG-PIT pilot corpus and the single-session part of the EMG-UKA corpus, just as for the baseline system. The phone-based recognizer is augmented with phonetic features with various weightings ranging from 0.00 (i.e. the PFs are not used) to 0.09. Note that these are per-feature weights, i.e. the *total* weight of the PFs ranges up to 0.72. Also, in order to make the training of the different recognizers comparable, the training data alignments which are iteratively computed by the Viterbi algorithm during train-

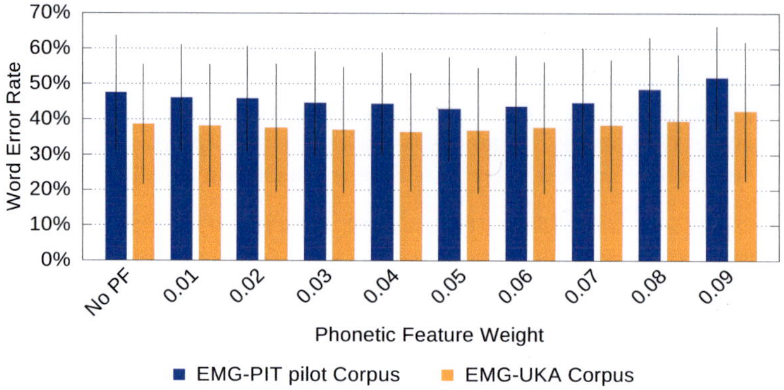

Figure 5.4 – WER for different weightings of the Phonetic Feature Streams, without Phonetic Feature bundling. Bars indicate standard deviation.

ing (see section 2.3.5) are based only on the phone stream, not on the PF streams; thus they are identical for all trained systems.

Figure 5.4 shows the results of these experiments. Clearly, PF modeling gives improvement, however raising the PF stream weight beyond about 0.05, which is a total PF weight of 0.40, causes the results to deteriorate. On the EMG-PIT pilot corpus, PF modeling with the PF streams weighted at 0.05 improves the WER from 47.47% for the phone-based system (compare table 4.1) to 42.96%, which is $\frac{47.47\%-42.96\%}{47.47\%} = 9.5\%$ relative; on the EMG-UKA corpus the improvement is from 38.55% WER to 36.83% WER, which is only 4.5% relative, albeit from a far better baseline. The observation that one cannot increase the PF stream weights beyond a certain threshold without causing accuracy deterioration confirms the results in [Kir99, Met05].

In order to establish the significance of the WER improvement, we performed recognition on the main part of the EMG-PIT corpus, i.e. on the evaluation set, using the optimal PF stream weighting of 0.05. From table 4.1, one sees that the phone system performs with 52.61% WER on this corpus. The PF-based system with a weighting of 0.05 per feature achieves 48.06% WER on average. The improvement is 8.65% relative, a result which is completely in accord with [Jou08].

We perform statistical validation by computing the *session-wise* improvement which PF modeling yields. The average absolute improvement per session is 4.55% with a 95% confidence interval ranging from 2.67% to 6.43%. From this result we conclude that the improvement is significantly above zero.

The multi-stream model is a realization of the third principle defined in section 5.1, i.e. data reuse. Indeed, the models in each stream are trained based on the *entire* training data set, where the feature extraction is not altered for different streams. Therefore, each feature frame is used nine times (once for the phone stream, once for each PF stream), and given that we do nothing more but using different partitionings of the training data, it is a remarkable success that this method yields a significant performance improvement.

5.2 Bundled Phonetic Features

This section describes the *phonetic feature bundling* algorithm, which is one of the central results of this thesis and a core component of the EMG-based Silent Speech Recognizer. We first presented this algorithm in [SW10].

5.2.1 Introduction and Motivation

First recall that it is intended to create a new modeling structure based on three principles: (1) Phonetic Feature modeling, (2) data-driven model optimization, and (3) data reuse. The last section 5.1.2 reports significant improvements by applying principles (1) and (3), but principle (2) has not yet been implemented.

A classical method to create optimized models in *acoustic* speech recognition is *context-dependent modeling*, see section 2.3.4, which is reported to yield WER improvements of up to almost 50% relative. How is this result achieved? The first key observation is that phone models should not be considered in isolation: Instead, the realization (i.e. the sound, or in the EMG case the articulator movements) of a phone depends on its neighboring phones (its "context"). This is accounted for by creating context-dependent models, where each phone depends on its left and right neighbor(s). Unfortunately this new structure implies that the number of trained unit models increases drastically, which is where the second key component of the algorithm comes into play: Phone contexts are automatically clustered according to a suitable similarity measure, so that the number of contexts which must be modeled is reduced.

In [WS09], we showed that context-dependent modeling significantly improves the WER of a speaker-independent EMG-based speech recognizer. However, this result does not transfer to session-dependent systems because the training data corpus is too small. We observed that the WER of the session-dependent recognizer increases when context-dependent modeling is used, and that the WER invariably gets worse when the number of context-dependent models is increased.

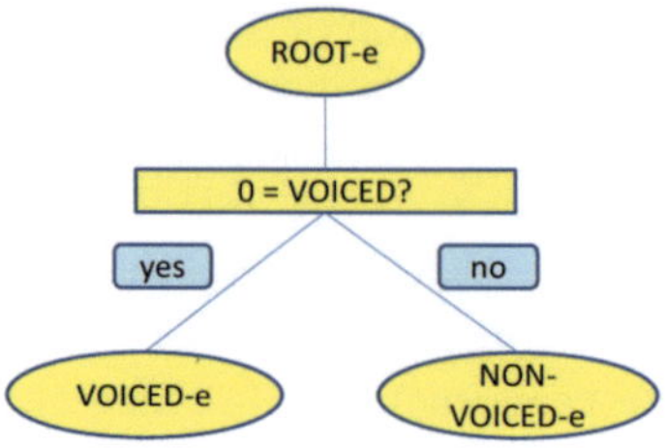

Figure 5.5 – Example of a partial PF tree (before PF bundling) for the VOICED stream. Only the "end" models, corresponding to the end part of the PF "VOICED", are shown. When a model for a specific phone is required, the algorithm traverses the tree, choosing the right branch by answering a *phonetic question*, e.g. for the phone [R], the question "0=VOICED?" (Is the current phone voiced?) is true, so the "VOICED-e" model would be used.

Context-dependent models are based on a refinement of context-independent phone models. The idea can be applied to our session-dependent EMG-based speech recognizers by changing the modeling paradigm: We start with the phonetic feature models from the previous section instead of phone models and then use decision-tree based model splitting to obtain more specific models. In the following paragraphs the algorithm is described in detail.

5.2.2 The PF Bundling Algorithm

Reconsider the multi-stream system as shown in figure 5.2. For PF bundling, each PF stream is considered *separately*, the phone stream is left unchanged.

According to the setup described in section 5.1, each stream comprises *seven* models, corresponding to the beginning, middle, or end of the present or absent phonetic feature, plus a special silence model. Note that the models for beginning, middle, and end of a PF are never combined (one might opt for a more general joint modeling of these substates, but we observed that this does not yield any benefit). In the remainder of this section, we call this model structure *unbundled PFs* for short.

The unbundled PF models may be implemented using a very simple phonetic decision tree, as shown in figure 5.5 using the "end" models of the "Voiced" stream as an example. Starting at the tree root, the phonetic question "0=VOICED" (Is the current phone voiced?) determines which model is to be used, based on the current phone.

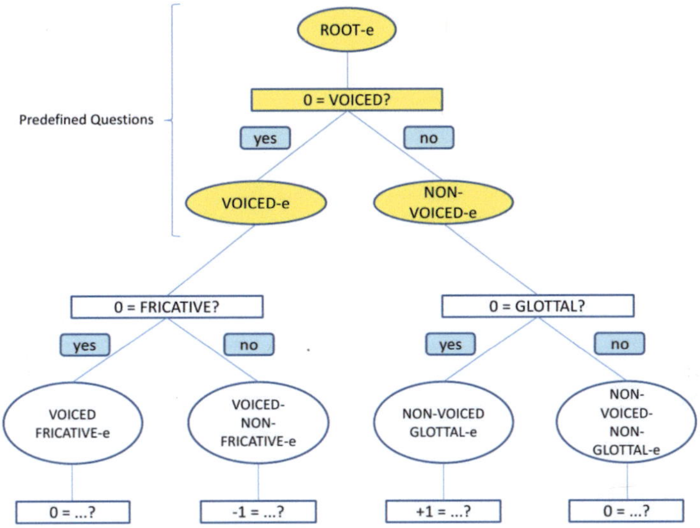

Figure 5.6 – Example of a partial BDPF tree for the VOICED stream. The upper nodes with yellow background are predefined and are also present when context-independent unbundled PFs are used (see figure 5.5); when BDPF models are used, the BDPF tree is generated from this basis. Questions ask for presence or absence of a PF in the current (0), preceding (-1), or following (+1) phone.

The purpose of phonetic feature bundling is to find an optimized model structure, balancing the requirement that there should not be too many different models (which would be difficult to properly estimate with a small training data corpus), and the requirement that the models should be fine-grained enough to capture the articulatory variability between different phones and phonetic features. A phonetic decision tree represents an *iterative* refinement of models, which makes it perfectly suited for balancing these requirements. In figure 5.6, it is shown how the basic phonetic decision tree is extended with more branchings based on phonetic feature questions, yielding models which correspond to "bundles" of phonetic features, e.g. "voiced fricative". The longer the paths in the tree are, the more specific the models become. At the bottom of the figure, questions like "-1=..." and "1=..." can be seen: By convention such formulas refer to the left or right context phone in an HMM, allowing the bundled PF models to incorporate context dependency.

The set of possible questions is predefined, it is based on questions for about 100 PFs. These PFs cover a large variety of subgroups of the IPA charts for vowels and consonants (see section 2.2.2), so we have rectified one problem of the unbundled PFs, namely that they do not allow discriminating all phones of the English language.

Each combination of a PF and a context position (-1, 0, 1) defines a question, figure 5.6 displays several examples. In addition, questions may be augmented by additionally asking whether the previous, current, or next phone is located at a word boundary. Due to the limited amount of training data, we do not consider larger context widths than ± 1, and in the experiments below, we allow the context questions to be suppressed altogether: this means that questions may only be asked for the *current* phone, and not for context phones. For the models which are created by this algorithm, we coined the name ***Bundled Phonetic Features*** (BDPF).

We remark that first results on applying the decision tree method with phonetic features (VOWEL and CONSONANT) as root nodes were already obtained for acoustic speech recognition in [YS03], albeit without using a multi-stream system. Only small WER improvements could be achieved, ranging around 3% relative, which is less than what we achieve with unbundled phonetic features. In section 5.2.3, we reconsider this system and give a possible explanation for this result.

In order to create a phonetic decision tree for any of the PF streams, the decision tree growing algorithm from [BdSG$^+$91] is performed, similar to the creation of context dependent models (see section 2.3.4):

1. Firstly, the algorithm is initialized with the set of six"unbundled" PF models representing the beginning, middle, and end of the respective present or absent phonetic feature, plus a silence model. These models are arranged into three decision trees, each like the one in figure 5.5, the silence model does not participate in the splitting process.
2. Now the recognizer with the "unbundled" PF models is trained according to the steps described in section 4.1.3. In particular, GMMs for the PF models are created, which is a requirement for choosing optimal model splits.
3. For each present or absent phonetic feature, all available phonetic contexts whose central phone matches the phonetic feature are collected (up to the predetermined maximal context width).
4. A new system is trained, having the following structure: the set of Gaussian component distributions remains unbundled. However, each phonetic context receives its *own* set of mixture weights. This is an example of *parameter tying*, balancing the requirements of fine granularity and trainability. In the context of phonetic decision tree growing, the important

property of the new modeling structure is that it yields a well-computable criterion for model splits.

5. In each step, *all* current leaf nodes and *all* possible questions are considered in order to determine the optimal split for this step (a minimum amount of training data is required for a node to participate in the splitting). The criterion for the optimal split is the loss of entropy in the mixture weights [FR97]: The entropy of the joint mixture weight distributions is subtracted from the entropy of the two resulting mixture weight distributions which will emerge if the split is performed. If this computation results in a high value, this means that the split will cause a high entropy loss, or information gain. Note that this only works because all phonetic contexts which match the same present or absent phonetic feature share the same Gaussian components, and that the computation is very quick, since the mixture weights just reflect the amount of training data samples for the underlying Gaussian components (compare equation 2.5), which is readily available.

6. The optimal split, which is the split which yields the highest entropy loss, is performed, thus creating two child nodes corresponding to BDPF models. The leaf node which was split is now a branching node in the decision tree.

7. Steps 5 and 6 are repeated until a termination criterion is met. In this study, the termination criterion is that a fixed number of leaves have been created, and we use the additional constraint that all nodes must receive enough training data. Further down, the effect of varying the termination criterion is investigated.

This algorithm is applied to all eight PF streams in the multi-stream framework. Finally, the recognizer is trained again, now using the newly created set of models. Note that we refrain from recomputing the LDA transformation, since we did not observe any benefit from this step. Training is performed according to the setup described in section 4.1.3, as usual: The GMM models are initialized with Merge-and-Split training, followed by four iterations of the Viterbi algorithm.

When PF bundling is performed, the original binary PF models are specialized more and more. During this process, BDPF models "converge" towards phone models, in the sense that a suitable series of phonetic questions uniquely determines a phone (e.g. in English, the description *unvoiced labiodental fricative* is only satisfied by the phone [f]). This is a key property of BDPF models: they are optimized models ranging between binary PF models, i.e. the most coarse possible model, and (context-dependent or context-independent) phone models, i.e. the most specialized possible model. The specialization is determined in a data-driven way, thus ensuring an optimal representation of the training data.

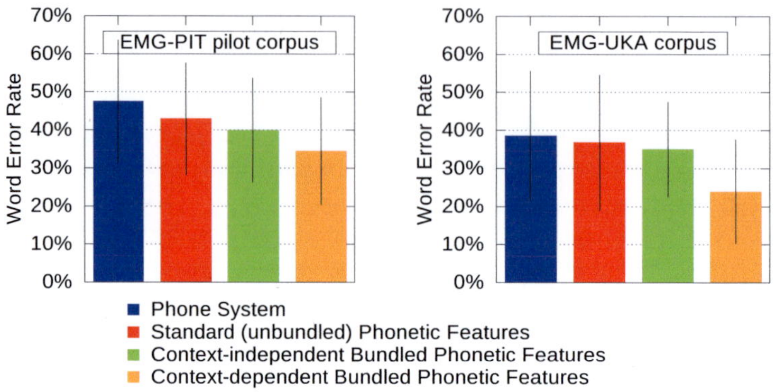

Figure 5.7 – Performance of Bundled Phonetic Features versus reference systems. Bars indicate standard deviation.

As an example for the usage of the BDPF models, assume that the VOICED stream with the PF tree shown in figure 5.6 needs to compute a score for the end part of the [r] phone of the word "true", consisting of the phone sequence [t] [r] [oo], and for a given feature vector. Computation is based on the PF tree in figure 5.6. Using a context width of one, the middle phone could be written as "R(T|OO)". Score computation starts at the tree root, and the context "R(T|OO)" is used to answer the question "Is the central phone voiced?" In this case the answer is "yes" since [r] is voiced, so we continue at the node "VOICED-e". The next question is "Is the central phone a fricative?". Since this is false, we now reach the node "VOICED NON-FRICATIVE-e" and continue accordingly, this time with a question about the left context phone [t] ("-1=..."), until a leaf node, corresponding to a trained GMM model, is reached.

5.2.3 Results and Analysis

Basic BDPF System For a first evaluation of the BDPF recognizer, we fix the following parameters:

- As in 5.1, eight PF streams are used, namely the ones corresponding to PFs which receive more than 1000 training data samples.
- The BDPF tree generation stops when 120 nodes are created, or when each node receives less than 50 training samples. Note that this criterion is evaluated *per stream*, so eventually, we will obtain $8 \cdot 120 = 960$ BDPF models.

System	EMG-PIT (pilot)		EMG-UKA	
	WER	rel. impr.	WER	rel. impr.
Phone-based (Baseline)	47.47%	-	38.55%	-
Unbundled PFs	42.96%	9.5%	36.83%	4.5%
Context-independent BDPFs	39.95%	15.8%	31.61%	8.1%
Context-dependent BDPFs	33.95%	28.5%	22.82%	40.8%

Table 5.1 – Summary of Word Error Rates of the Phonetic Feature systems. Relative improvement are *towards the phone-based baseline system.*

- We consider both the *context-independent* system (i.e. the system where phonetic questions about the left and right contexts are *not* allowed) and the fully *context-dependent* BDPF system with a maximal context of ± 1.

Later on, we will show that these parameters are optimal. The feature extraction is taken from the baseline system: We use the TD10 feature, and we use the 12 most discriminant dimensions after LDA. As described above, LDA is computed on the context-independent phones; we also performed experiments on recomputing the LDA for each PF stream, but did not observe substantial improvement from this step.

Figure 5.7 and table 5.1 show the Word Error Rates of the following four recognizers: the standard phone-based recognizer, the recognizer with "unbundled" phonetic features and optimal settings from section 5.1.3, and the context-independent and context-dependent BDPF recognizer. The result clearly shows that BDPF modeling yields a substantially improved accuracy: On the EMG-PIT corpus, the average WER decreases from 42.96% for unbundled PFs to 33.95% for the context-dependent BDPF system, which is a relative improvement of 21.0%. Compared to the phone-based system with 47.47% WER, the relative improvement is 28.5%. On the EMG-UKA corpus, the WER drops from 36.83% for unbundled PFs to 22.82% for context-dependent BDPFs, which is an improvement of 38.0%. The context-dependent BDPF system yields a relative improvement over the phone-based system of more than 40%.

The context-independent BDPFs also perform well, with 7.0% resp. 14.2% relative improvement towards unbundled PFs and 15.8% resp. 8.1% relative improvement towards the phone-based system. However, this improvement is not consistent, for some sessions we actually observe that the WER rises when context-independent PF bundling is applied.

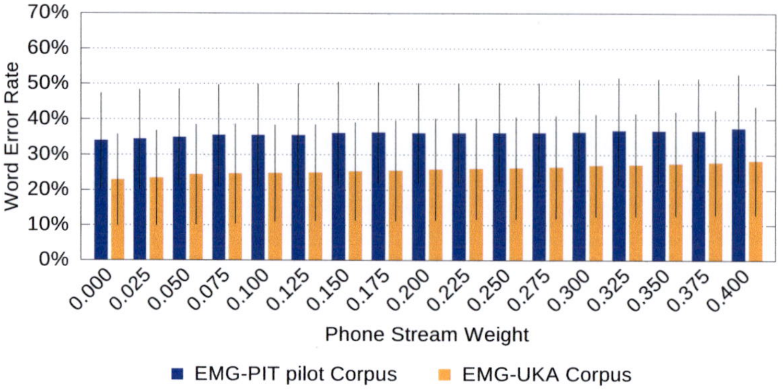

Figure 5.8 – Performance of the context-dependent BDPF System with different weightings of the phone stream. Bars indicate standard deviation.

System Optimization In this section, the aspect of parameter optimization is discussed. As in section 4.3, optimization is performed with a focus on understanding properties of the system, rather than tuning the system for maximal performance. Note that all following experiments are based on the context-dependent BDPF system, i.e. questions for the left and right phone context are allowed in the decision tree creation stage.

As a first step, we ask how much the phone stream needs to contribute when BDPF streams are used. For this experiment, we retain the constraint from section 5.1.2 that all BDPF streams must have the same weight. The phone stream weight is varied from 0.0 to 0.4. The Word Error Rates obtained with these experiments are displayed in figure 5.8: Increasing the phone stream weight causes an almost linear rise of the WER on both the EMG-PIT (pilot) and the EMG-UKA corpus. We note that the variance between sessions is large, for example, on the sole session of speaker 5 of the EMG-UKA corpus, the WER falls from 35.40% to 30.30% when the phone stream weight is increased from 0 to 0.025. In contrast, on session 2 of speaker 1 we achieve a WER of 34.30% without phone stream and 42.40% with a phone stream weight on 0.025. For the vast majority of sessions, using the phone stream, even with a very low weight, causes declining accuracy. From the observations, we conclude that the overall best system is achieved *without* the phone stream, and all further experiments are therefore based on the BDPF streams alone.

The next experiment answers the question how many BDPF streams are required for optimal recognition performance, and how the performance of the recognizer changes when the number of streams is varied. In section 5.2, we argued for

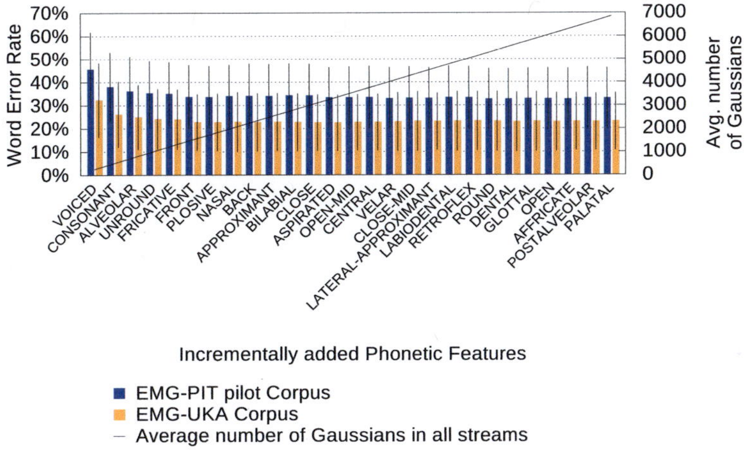

Figure 5.9 – Performance of the context-dependent BDPF System with different numbers of streams for testing, and average number of Gaussians in the systems. Streams are incrementally added according to the sorting on the horizontal axis. Bars indicate standard deviation.

using eight streams, but under very different conditions. In those experiments *unbundled* PFs were used, where the streams each have very different properties in terms of available training data for the models for present and absent PFs, and in terms of the encoded information.

So for the following experiment, phonetic decision trees and BDPF models for 27 BDPF streams were trained, corresponding to the 27 most frequent PFs in our setup, omitting redundant PFs. For testing, streams were incrementally added in order of PF frequency, so the first eight streams correspond to the standard streams chosen in section 5.1.2. The total weight of 1.0 was split equally across all PF streams, the phone stream was never used.

In figure 5.9 the result of this experiment is charted: It is clearly visible that only the first five or so streams contribute to the improvement of the recognition result. After this, the system neither improves nor degrades. The latter is remarkable since e.g. for the PF "PALATAL", only 100 training data samples are present (see figure 5.3), but the explanation is simple: Both the models for a present and absent phonetic feature are part of the corresponding PF stream and participate in splitting.

Since the model splits depend on the available amount of training data, it is clear that for a stream where the present PF receives little training data, most splits are performed on models for the absent phonetic feature. In the most extreme case, there exist sessions where e.g. the set of BDPF models for the PALATAL stream consist of three unsplit models for the substates (beginning, middle, and end) of the PALATAL feature, and for all other BDPFs in this stream, the PALATAL feature is *not* present. Additionally, for example the PALATAL stream, being the 27th stream to be added, of course only contributes to the total score with a weight of $1/27 \approx 4\%$, so a major influence on the result cannot be expected.

Figure 5.9 additionally plots the average number of Gaussians, i.e. the model size, summed over all contributing streams, and averaged over all sessions and speakers. We see that with an increasing number of BDPF streams, the system size grows linearly: each BDPF stream, independent of its root phonetic feature, comprises a similar number of Gaussian models. This result is very consistent across speakers.

A major observation taken from figure 5.9 is that using just one, or even two streams, is not enough to unleash the full potential of the BDPF models: around five streams are required. This may partially explain the small WER improvement of Yu and colleagues [YS03], who create a decision tree similar to the ones employed in this study in an acoustic speech recognition scenario, obtaining only a small improvement (up to 3% relative). In that work, only a single knowledge stream, corresponding to a single phonetic decision tree, is used, whereas our study is firmly based on the multi-stream scenario. Another explanation may be that the corpus used in [YS03] is far larger than our EMG-PIT and EMG-UKA corpora (up to 160 hours of speech training data). It is expected that on such a large corpus, classical context-dependent models would also perform well, so that the BDPF modeling yields only a small improvement. This result underlines the importance of BDPF modeling, which brings flexible, optimized models to comparatively small data corpora.

We ran additional experiments on varying the relative weighting of the BDPF streams according to a discriminative criterion (Discriminative Model Combination (DMC) [Bey00]). However, no consistent performance improvement or degradation was obtained by using DMC (additionally, the computation time for model training rose drastically). We propose that this is due to the fact that the BDPF streams *converge* when the phonetic decision tree is large enough: a split which is important in one stream is expected to occur at some point in any other stream, too. This means that the PF streams have similar discriminative power. In the following we quantify this statement, showing that it is indeed true as long as *multiple* streams are used. In order to gain insight into the discriminative power of the BDPF streams, we ran the following experiment. We trained 10 context-dependent BDPF streams, in the order depicted in figure 5.9 (the limit

Number (n) of BDPF streams	Non-discriminable phone pairs	
	EMG-PIT pilot Corpus	EMG-UKA Corpus
1	74.9 ± 34.8	83.5 ± 59.3
2	29.6 ± 13.7	32.7 ± 26.9
3	16.7 ± 8.5	18.4 ± 14.6
4	11.0 ± 5.7	12.4 ± 9.1
5	7.8 ± 4.1	9.2 ± 6.2
6	5.9 ± 3.2	7.2 ± 4.5
7	4.6 ± 2.5	5.9 ± 3.5
8	3.6 ± 2.0	4.9 ± 2.8
9	2.9 ± 1.6	4.2 ± 2.2
10	2.4 ± 1.2	3.6 ± 1.8

Table 5.2 – Number of non-discriminable phone pairs with different numbers of BDPF streams (mean and standard deviation). The values are averaged over all n-tuples of BDPF streams. See text for details.

of 10 streams was chosen to keep the computation time under control). Then we considered *all* n-tuples of distinct streams, for $n = 1, \dots, 10$.

For each such tuple, we determined how many *pairs of phones* could be discriminated based on these streams. For simplicity, only the phonetic decision trees for the middle subphone were considered. A phone pair is said to be discriminable if *at least one* BDPF stream groups these two phones into different categories, i.e. decision tree leaves. Clearly, the more BDPF streams there are, the more phone pairs can be discriminated.

In order to keep the experiment simple, we did not consider phone contexts in this experiment, and we likewise disregarded the word boundary tag, which additionally serves to discriminate models (see the description in section 5.2.2). Since we use 47 phones for the decision trees (45 "true" phones, a silence phone, and a special padding phone for unknown contexts), we obtain $\frac{47 \cdot 46}{2} = 1081$ phone pairs.

The average and standard deviation of the count of nondiscriminable phone pairs for different numbers of BDPF streams is shown in table 5.2. The average was taken over all possible tuples of BDPF streams and all sessions of the respective corpus. It can be seen that with only one BDPF stream, a large number of phone pairs (84 resp. 74 on average) cannot be discriminated. With more streams, the number of nondiscriminable phone pairs falls drastically. This corresponds well with the result from figure 5.9, where we observed that one BDPF stream alone does not yield good recognition results, but that just a few more streams suffice to attain optimal performance.

When we use eight BDPF streams, there are around 3 – 5 phone pairs on average which are never discriminated. Some of these pairs are irrelevant in the classification process, for example, if one of the phones is the special padding phone. Beyond this, typical non-discriminable pairs include phones which only contrast by voicedness, as well as phone pairs whose pronunciations are very similar. The latter is true for some vowel contrasts, e.g. a typical nondiscriminable phone pair comprises the two different phones for the 'oo' vowels in the English words "do" and "hood".

This result matches the assumptions we made on the process of EMG-based speech recognition (see section 4.4): In particular, phones where articulator movements are very similar may be hard to discriminate. We also note that the number of nondiscriminable phone pairs is consistently lower for the EMG-PIT corpus than for the EMG-UKA corpus, even though the WER on the EMG-PIT corpus is higher: This might be due to pronunciation mistakes by the non-native speakers who recorded the EMG-UKA corpus, however, so far we do not have any proof for this hypothesis.

Finally, we relate the number of nondiscriminable phone pairs to the Word Error Rates of the EMG-based speech recognizer. For each session of the pilot part of the EMG-PIT corpus and the EMG-UKA corpus, we consider the WER for $n = 1, \ldots, 27$ BDPF streams, and we compute the number of nondiscriminable phone pairs with $n = 1, \ldots, 27$ BDPF streams. For this experiment, the streams are always considered in the standard ordering, as shown in figure 5.9.

We observe a relation between the WER and the number of nondiscriminable phone pairs: Averaged over all sessions, the WER and the number of nondiscriminable phone pairs correlate with a correlation coefficient of 0.51 on the EMG-UKA corpus and 0.66 on the EMG-PIT pilot corpus. So we see that there is a relation between lack of phone discrimination and Word Error Rate.

From the results of the phone discrimination experiments we draw two conclusions. First, we see that adding more streams brings a different model structure, but beyond five streams or so, hardly more discriminative power is gained. Therefore we *fix the number of BDPF streams* which are used in all future experiments to eight streams, based on the PF streams which were also used in the unbundled case: This allows comparison of the unbundled and bundled PF setups, yields optimal results, and avoids unnecessary computations.

Second, table 5.2 asserts that over all sessions and *all possible combinations* of eight BDPF streams, the number of nondiscriminable phone pairs remains quite stable (the standard deviation is small). Thus is does not matter very much which set of BDPF streams is used, as long as there are enough different ones. This finally proves our assertion stated above that BDPF streams indeed have similar

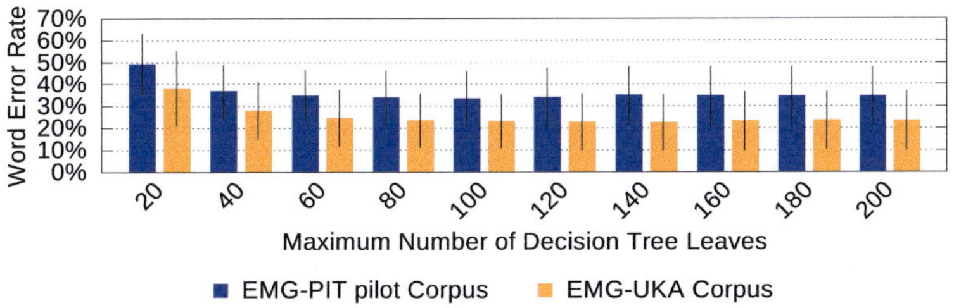

Figure 5.10 – Performance of the context-dependent BDPF System with different decision tree size limits. Bars indicate standard deviation.

discriminative power, *as long as several ones are used.* However, if we consider just one stream, we take from table 5.2 that the amount of nondiscriminable phones varies quite drastically: So the *single* BDPF streams appear to differ in their discrimination capabilities.

The last parameter optimization relates to the decision tree creation process. So far, the stopping criterion for the decision tree creation was the fixed number of 120 leaves, or that no current leaf node received enough training data to allow a split. Figure 5.10 shows the performance of the recognizer when the maximum number of leaves is varied: The optimum for the EMG-PIT corpus is 100 leaves, for the EMG-UKA corpus, the optimum is reached at 140 leaves, however beyond 80, the differences are insignificant. At higher numbers, the results do not change any more, since in this case, there is not enough data per node to continue splitting, so the process stops early and the maximum number of tree leaves is not reached: Our experiments show that the number of actually created leaves is bounded at around 140 – 160, averaged over all trees. When lower thresholds than 140 leaves are used, the maximum number of leaves is almost always reached.

We also varied the minimum amount of training data required for splitting a node and found similar results: Within a broad range, varying the stopping criterion for the decision tree split does not yield significant changes. For this reason we refrained from evaluating other stopping criteria for the decision tree splitting. For all further experiments in this thesis, the number of 120 leaves per decision tree was chosen as the average between the optima on the two corpora.

Significance of the Results In order to validate the results obtained within this chapter, experiments were performed on the evaluation data set, i.e. the main part of the EMG-PIT corpus. The following hypotheses are to be checked: First,

System	WER	rel. impr.	abs. impr. with conf.
Phone-based (Baseline)	52.6%	-	-
Unbundled PFs	48.1%	8.6%	4.5% ± 1.88%
Context-independent BDPFs	45.2%	6.0%	2.9% ± 1.90%
Context-dependent BDPFs	35.7%	21.0%	9.5% ± 1.85%

Table 5.3 – Word Error Rates of the different PF systems on the evaluation set (EMG-PIT main corpus), with relative improvements and *absolute* improvements with confidence intervals.

we wish to assert that the improvement from the phone-based baseline system to the unbundled PF system is significant. This would confirm the results from [Jou08] on a new corpus. Second, we claim that context-independent BDPF modeling yields significantly reduced WERs compared to unbundled PFs. Third, we claim that allowing context questions in the BDPF creation process yields another significant improvement. All experiments are performed with the respective optimal parameter settings.

The results on the evaluation corpus are summarized in table 5.3. For each system, we give the absolute and relative improvements towards the previous system, for the absolute improvements, we computed 95% confidence intervals. All confidence intervals have lower boundaries well above zero, so we conclude that all improvements are statistically significant. The relative improvement of the context-dependent BDPFs towards the phone-based baseline system is 32.1%—this is in line with the results on the development corpora, on the EMG-PIT pilot corpus, we achieved 28.5% relative improvement, on the EMG-UKA corpus, the relative improvement was 40.8%. The large variation between the corpora reflects the large variation between the results for different speakers, which we already reported in section 4.2.

5.3 Summary

This chapter introduced *Bundled Phonetic Features* (BDPF) as the basic modeling unit for the EMG-based speech recognizer. The BDPFs are used within a *multi-stream* framework, which is a major prerequisite for their effectiveness.

The modeling structure is based on three prinicples, namely Phonetic Feature modeling, optimized models, and data reuse, where the PF bundling algorithm creates optimized models, and the multi-stream framework is a powerful method for data reuse. The key property of the BDPFs is that they represent optimal models ranging between binary PF models and phone models (with or without context dependency), i.e. between very general and very specific models, and that the optimization is performed in a data-driven way, with the target criterion of optimizing the representation of the training data. Now that a robust and powerful modeling structure for our EMG-based speech recognition systems has been established, future work might include investigation of discriminative criteria for the decision tree creation (e.g. [WHNT+10]), as well as standard discriminative training methods, however this is beyond the scope of this thesis.

Chapter 6

Recognition Across Different Speaking Modes

This chapter deals with EMG-based speech recognition across different speaking modes, which comprise normally spoken, whispered, and silently mouthed speech. We review the mechanism of articulation control; this serves as a basis for the discussion of speaking mode discrepancies, and helps explaining some of the observations presented in this chapter. Recognition results on cross-mode and multi-mode systems, which cover several speaking modes in training and testing, are presented, tackling the problem of accurately bootstrapping a silent speech recognizer. Finally, the discrepancy between speaking modes is analyzed both at model level and signal level, giving rise to the key result of this chapter: The ***Spectral Mapping*** *algorithm, a signal-based adaptation method to compensate for the difference between the EMG signals of audible and silent speech, reduces the Word Error Rate by up to 11.5% relative.*

The experiments presented so far were performed only on EMG signals of *audible* speech (audible EMG). Since the key purpose of the EMG-based speech recognizer is the recognition of *silent* speech, this chapter deals with EMG-based speech recognition across different *speaking modes*. The experiments show that discrepancies between these speaking modes exist, and it is the purpose of this chapter to present means of analyzing and coping with them. Speaking modes include audible (normally spoken), whispered, and silently mouthed speech, they are defined in section 2.2.3. We call the corresponding EMG recordings of speech *audible EMG*, *whispered EMG*, and *silent EMG*, respectively.

This chapter is structured as follows. We begin with a review of the process of articulatory control: How does the brain generate the complex muscular activation patterns which are needed to produce intelligible speech? To answer this question, a well-known contemporary model, the DIVA model [GGT06], is presented. The question of articulatory control is clearly important in all fields of speech-related research, but we consider it particularly important in this chapter since in silent speech, a very important component of the articulation process, namely the *acoustic feedback* which stems from a speaker hearing his or her own voice, is missing. We propose that the speaking mode discrepancies described in this chapter are partly caused by the lack of acoustic feedback.

The experimental section of this chapter starts with the introduction of *cross-mode* and *multi-mode* recognition systems. Here the term "cross-mode" indicates that training and testing are performed on data from different speaking modes. "Multi-mode" refers to systems where training is performed on data from more than one speaking mode. Consequently, a system which uses the same speaking mode for training and testing is called a "single-mode" system. Results are presented on cross-mode and multi-mode systems with whispered EMG and silent EMG.

Based on the multi-mode systems, we focus on silent speech and analyze the discrepancy between the audible and silent speaking modes. For this purpose, model-based methods and signal-based methods are devised. From a signal-based discrepancy measure, the *PSD ratio*, we deduce the *Spectral Mapping* algorithm, a signal-based adaptation method crafted to make EMG signals of audible and silent speech more similar. It is shown that spectral mapping improves the cross-mode recognition of silent EMG by up to 11.5% relative, the multi-mode systems improve by up to 11.4% relative when applied to silent EMG.

All experiments presented in this chapter are performed with the session-dependent BDPF-based recognizer presented in chapter 5, using optimal settings. We use the EMG-PIT corpus and the multi-mode part of the EMG-UKA corpus, as before, the main part of the EMG-PIT corpus is used for final statistical evaluation. Note that for all systems, results between different speaking modes are directly comparable, since recordings of different speaking modes use the same set of sentences (see section 3.2). This chapter in based on our publications [JWS10a, JWS10b, WJS11, WJS12, WJS14].

6.1 Controlling the Articulatory Apparatus

Figure 3.1 shows an overview of the facial muscles. The facial muscles move the articulators, which include the lips, jaw, tongue, etc. The position of the articulators in turn determines which phone is produced. The generation and classification of speech sounds is described in section 2.2, it can be observed that the established phonetic categories, e.g. the vowel quadrangle or the consonant features *manner* and *position*, are based on articulator configuration and positions.

However, controlling the articulators in actual speech is a complex process:

- Each phone is created by the movements of multiple articulators
- The problem of determining articulator trajectories for a given phone sequence is ill-posed, i.e. multiple solutions exist [RKT03]
- Each articulator may be affected by various muscles, and these muscles need very precise control in order to achieve the desired result
- In continuous speech, sounds may be altered or suppressed, and *coarticulation* causes blurring between adjacent phones. Still, the produced speech remains understandable, which requires a high amount of fine-tuning (and the help of the listener).

Furthermore, humans are able to produce speech under a variety of constraints and conditions, which have to be compensated for. This includes artificial constraints (e.g. when a bite block is inserted into the mouth), but also applies to adolescent persons, where the size and properties of the articulators change over time. Humans can also adapt to deficiencies on the listeners side (e.g. we speak more clearly if the listener has hearing difficulties).

So far, there is no method to fully measure or visualize the processes which occur in the human brain during speech production. Instead, several *models* have been developed to explain properties of human speech. Here one well-known model is presented, namely the DIVA model, which was developed by Frank H. Guenther and colleagues at Boston University[1] [GGT06] and is considered one of the leading approaches in the field.

DIVA (Directions Into Velocities of Articulators) covers a range of phenomena which are observed in speech production and learning. It is a neurocomputational model, thus it provides theoretical explanations about processes in the human brain, but also allows computational simulation. The key components of

[1]Resources on the DIVA model are found at `http://www.bu.edu/speechlab/research/the-diva-model`

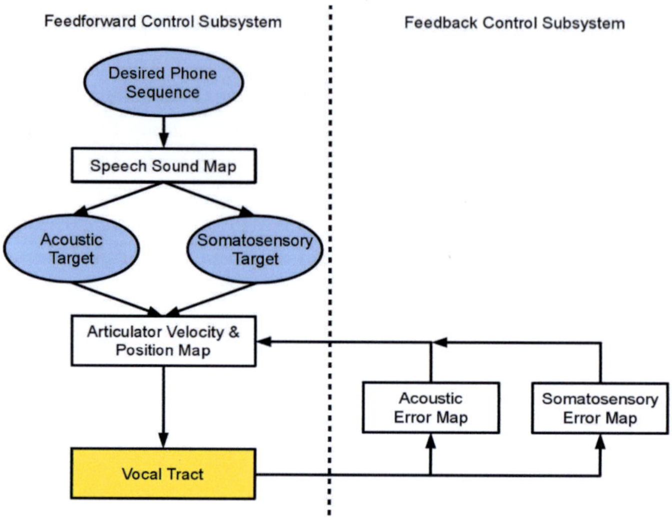

Figure 6.1 – Simplified DIVA model chart following [GGT06, figure 1]. The white rectangles correspond to component neural networks.

the model are several neural networks whose interplay maps target phone sequences into velocities of articulators. The articulatory trajectories are passed on to a simulated vocal tract.

The DIVA neural networks represent parts of the articulation process. A key feature is *control*: Articulator positions are controlled by the feedforward control subsystem, and acoustic and somatosensory feedback from the articulation process affect the articulation via the feedback control subsystem. Figure 6.1 shows a simplified chart of the DIVA model (compare [GGT06, figure 1]).

There exists a relationship between the DIVA model and the human brain which is well-supported by experimental observation. In particular, some of the components shown in figure 6.1 can be identified in human brain anatomy, for example, the *Articulator Velocity and Position Map* corresponds to the motor cortex (see section 2.1). Such results suggest that important conclusions about human speech production can be drawn from the DIVA model, even though it might be very hard to prove that *all* its parts accurately reflect the speech production process.

From figure 6.1, it can be seen that the DIVA model contains two *targets* for the articulation process, which are used for both feedforward and feedback control, namely the *acoustic* and the *somatosensory* targets. The acoustic target essentially describes the sound of a speech unit, the somatosensory target relates to the tactile perception which is associated with a speech segment. The DIVA neural networks learn how to create sounds which realize these targets [Gue95], see below; when DIVA has been trained, the model can generate speech from a target phone sequence, *and* it can regenerate an acoustic speech fragment which is played to it—this underlines that the DIVA neural networks are substantially more versatile than mere feed-forward networks.

The existence of the acoustic target suggests that at the brain level, knowledge about the desired acoustic representation of a sound is used, and that this knowledge is only mapped to articulator trajectories at a later stage. Also, the acoustic targets in the feedback subsystem indicates that the process of speech generation will be severely affected when acoustic feedback fails, as is the case for silent speech. The existence of the somatosensory target indicates the importance of tactile perception in speech production.

Speech sound generation starts at the *Speech Sound Map*. It encodes frequent speech sounds of the target language, where according to [GGT06], a speech sound may be "a phoneme, syllable, word, or short phrase that is frequently encountered in the native language and therefore has associated with it a stored motor program for its production." So we see that speech sounds within the DIVA framework are defined more liberally than in typical speech recognition systems, which use a rather rigid structure (see section 2.3).

Common speech sounds are triggered by the activation of single neurons in the input layer of the speech sound map. Uncommon phonetic sequences are not represented in this way, instead, if they are to be articulated, they must be composed out of smaller units. The set of speech sounds is not hard-coded in the DIVA neural network, instead, it must be generated during training.

Beginning at the speech sound map, the articulation process follows a feedforward pattern. The speech sound map encodes acoustic and somatosensory target regions (see [Gue95] for details about these target regions), which influence the articulator velocity and position map: Here the conversion of desired speech sounds into articulatory movements takes place. Finally, the output of this map controls a simulated vocal tract (according to [GGT06], the current implementation of the DIVA model uses a modified version of the synthesizer described in [Mae90]). Thus the output layer of the articulator velocity and position map reflects the degrees of freedom of the articulation process, for example, the raising or lowering of jaw or lips, and the multiple possible movements for the tongue; see [Gue95, table 3] for a complete summary. During articulation, feedback is collected and fed into the acoustic and somatosensory error maps, which in turn influence the articulator velocity and position map and thus correct articulation errors.

Training of the DIVA model is based on a *babbling phase*, during which random articulatory movements are produced. These movements create acoustic and somatosensory feedback, which are used to train the neural connections within the DIVA component networks. The tuning of the neural network, based on the randomly generated data, uses standard algorithmic methods and is (shortly) described in [GGT06, Appendix B]. However, it should be noted that this training is "self-organized" in the sense that "there are no 'training sets' for the system's mappings as in standard backpropagation algorithms" [Gue95, Section 1].

It is of great interest how the *structure* of the neural networks, in particular the topology of the speech sound map input layer, emerges. While the topology of the output layer is determined by the degrees of freedom of the simulated vocal tract, the input layer of the speech sound map, encoding the set of "common" speech sounds, is undefined at first. It is tuned *after* the babbling phase, the process works by playing training samples to the model and simultaneously activating the corresponding neuron of the speech sound map, see [GGT06, Section 6] for details.

This training phase is notable since it resembles the way an infant is assumed to acquire speech skills, namely, by hearing the speech of other persons, and trying to reproduce it [GGT06, Section 6]. At first, the "babbling" of a small child only produces isolated phones or syllables, quite different from adult speech; during the development of the child's cognitive and physiological abilities, more and more complex speech sounds are generated [Gue95, Section 2.1].

This final issue touches the question how complex structures in the brain are built up during infancy. There exist several studies (not all related to the DIVA model), which hypothesize that indeed, the speech sound map input layer has a physical representation in the human brain: Single neurons which may be activated in order to generate particular speech sounds actually exist [KKU$^+$02]. These neurons are assumed to have similar properties as the famous *mirror neurons* [RC04]: Mirror neurons in the brains of humans and certain animals are active when any kind of action is performed *or* observed: Thus they are said to be the foundation of learning by imitation, which is a major human capability, as well as of human social behavior. Regarding the process of speech skill acquisition, it is assumed that the input layer of the speech sound map is formed by neurons which functionally correspond to such mirror neurons [GGT06, Section 3.1]. [RC04] uses the formulation that humans might "possess an echo-neuron system [...] that motorically 'resonates' when the individual listens to verbal material". This might explain how children learn how to speak, and how they quickly adapt to the language(s) they hear during early childhood.

Here we conclude the overview of the DIVA model, of course, many details cannot be reported here due to space limitations. A central property of the model is the relevance of high-level acoustic (auditory) and somatosensory (tactile) targets for speech production, rather than articulatory targets.

This has got an important consequence for the experiments on Silent Speech conducted in this thesis: it becomes clear that lack of acoustic feedback, which occurs during production of Silent Speech, impacts the production of speech, and thus the articulatory movements. This is empirically verified by the deteriorating articulation accuracy of hearing-impaired persons [OM82], see section 2.2.3.

The lack of acoustic feedback, but also the articulation differences between audible and silent speech (see section 2.2.3), are expected to manifest as a discrepancy between the EMG signals of these speaking modes. This is clearly a detriment when building a silent speech recognizer, on the other hand, EMG can be used as a research tool to study silent articulation.

6.2 Recognition of Whispered Speech

6.2.1 Single-Mode Training

As a first step towards multi-mode EMG-based speech recognition, we investigate how our recognizer deals with EMG signals of *whispered* speech, i.e. whispered EMG. We only use the multi-mode part of the EMG-UKA corpus, since the EMG-PIT corpus does not contain recordings of whispered speech.

For training a recognizer on whispered EMG, we apply the BDPF-based recognizer just as for audible EMG, using the optimal parameters from section 5.2.3. Since parallely recorded acoustic data for whispered speech is available, we used standard *label bootstrapping* for initialization, as described in section 4.1.1: We manually checked some of the generated time-alignments and found them reasonably accurate, despite the fact that the underlying BN speech recognizer was trained on normally spoken speech.

Four experiments are performed, resulting from different combinations of training and test data: We train our recognizer either on audible or on whispered EMG, and likewise, we test the recognizer on audible or on whispered EMG. This is denoted as follows: for example, a system trained on whispered EMG and tested on audible EMG is marked by "Whis $\rightarrow$ Aud".

The results are charted in figure 6.2: Blue bars show recognition results on audible EMG, orange bars show recognition results on whispered EMG, and the

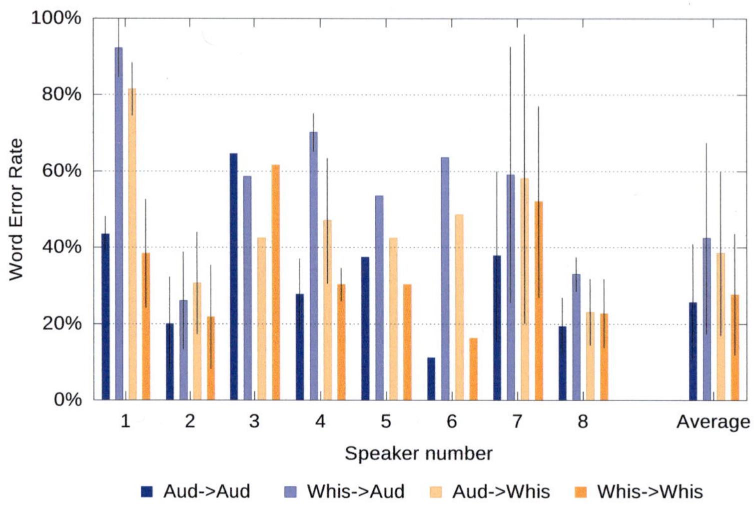

Figure 6.2 – Speaker breakdown of Word Error Rates for audible and *whispered* speech on the EMG-UKA corpus. The label A $\rightarrow$ B means that the recognizer was trained on speaking mode A and tested on speaking mode B. Bars indicate standard deviation.

semi-transparent bars indicate the results on cross-mode systems, i.e. Aud $\rightarrow$ Whis and Whis $\rightarrow$ Aud. Note that the Aud $\rightarrow$ Aud system is identical to the optimal system from the last chapter 5, however the average WER given here is different since we only use the multi-mode subset of the EMG-UKA corpus, instead of its whole audible part.

It can be observed that for all speakers, the WERs for both single-mode systems are within the same range, indicating that whispered speech is recognized as well as audible speech. Surprisingly, the WER on the cross-mode systems frequently increases, sometimes dramatically: This indicates that the articulator activity is different for audible and whispered speech, and that the extent of this difference is very much speaker-dependent. The worst cross-mode results are observed for speaker 1; for speakers 2 and 8, it can be seen that the loss of accuracy for the cross-mode systems is lower than for the other speakers. In the EMG-UKA corpus, speakers 2 and 8 are the most experienced speakers, i.e. the speakers with the largest number of recording sessions, so it can be assumed that practice improves the consistency of speech across different speaking modes. On the other hand, during recording it was observed that speaker 1 found consistent

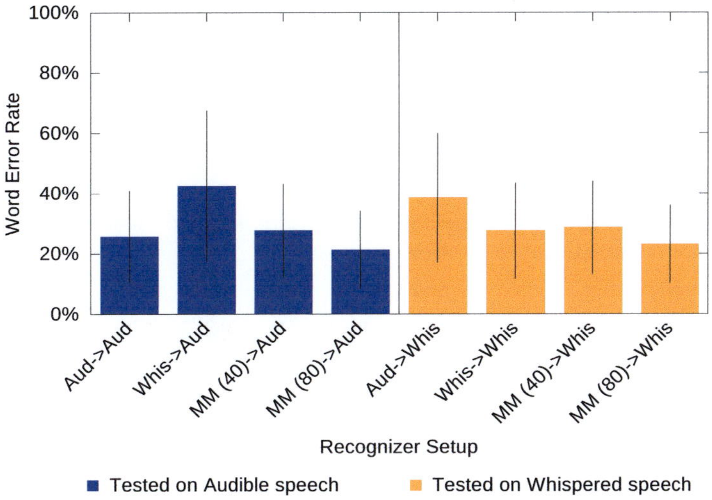

Figure 6.3 – Average Word Error Rates on audible and whispered speech, for single-mode, cross-mode, and multi-mode (MM) training. The number in parentheses stands for the number of training sentences on the multi-mode systems. Bars indicate standard deviation.

whispering very difficult, so the high WER of this speaker across speaking modes might also be attributed to incorrect articulation.

6.2.2 Multi-Mode Training

As a second experiment, we train multi-mode (MM) systems on training data from both the audible and whispered speaking mode. This allows us to train systems on 80 training sentences, which is twice as much as for the single-session systems. For comparison, we report results for multi-mode systems trained on 40 training sentences as well: For this purpose we split our training database, so that the 40 multi-mode training sentences are assured to have different textual content. The 80-sentence systems are expected to perform better than the 40-sentence systems due to the increased amount of training data.

Figure 6.3 shows that this is indeed the case. First, we observe that the multi-mode systems trained with 40 training sentences perform only slightly worse than the single-mode systems, and substantially better than the cross-mode systems. This indicates that while audible EMG and whispered EMG are different, they well complement each other. This is reconfirmed by the experiments on

Train \ Test	Audible EMG	Whispered EMG
Audible EMG	25.7%	38.5%
Whispered EMG	42.5%	27.7%
Multi-Mode (40 sent.)	27.7%	28.7%
Multi-Mode (80 sent.)	21.5%	23.1%

Table 6.1 – Summary of Word Error Rates for single-mode, cross-mode, and multi-mode training with audible and whispered EMG

80 training sentences from the audible and whispered speaking modes: Here the results are substantially better than on the single-mode systems. Table 6.1 summarizes the results of the experiments on whispered EMG.

This result is relevant because it is a design goal of EMG-based speech recognizers to allow seamless switching between different speaking modes. While speaking mode awareness might be achieved by using single-mode recognizers and detecting the current speaking mode prior to the main recognition process, we believe this method to be cumbersome and error-prone. In contrast, a recognizer which provides out-of-the-box recognition of EMG data with multiple speaking modes offers far greater flexibility. Additionally, speaking mode boundaries might not always be well-defined: Whispered speech, as an example, may range from a "stage whisper" to very quiet, almost inaudible speech, and during silent articulation certain phones, e.g. plosives, might still be heard, see section 2.2.3.

6.3 Recognition of Silent Speech

6.3.1 Single-Mode Training

When we intend to train a recognizer for *silent* EMG in the same way as the recognizers for audible or whispered EMG were trained, we encounter the problem that acoustic-generated labels, which are necessary for bootstrapping the recognizer (see section 4.1.1), are not available. In [WJTS09], we devised two methods for training a recognizer for silent EMG: The *Cross-Modal testing* approach means that a recognizer is trained on audible EMG data and tested on silent EMG data. *Cross-Modal labeling* means that time-alignments ("labels") for the silent EMG data are computed by forced-aligning the EMG data with a recognizer previously trained on audible EMG. These labels are used for training specific models for silent EMG, or for training a multi-mode recognizer.

These methods are easily integrated into the framework used in this thesis. Assuming that session-dependent recognizers for audible EMG are available, the silent EMG time-alignments are computed, after which silent EMG can be used for training just like audible and whispered EMG. We now perform similar experiments as in the last section, namely, we train our recognizer either on audible or on silent EMG, and likewise, we test the recognizer on audible or on silent EMG. Figure 6.4 shows a speaker breakdown of the results of these experiments for both the EMG-PIT pilot corpus and the EMG-UKA corpus, using the same notation as above, e.g. "Sil → Aud" means that a system is trained on silent EMG and tested on audible EMG.

It can be observed that generally, the WER for silent EMG is notably higher than for audible EMG. On the EMG-UKA corpus, audible EMG is recognized with 25.7% WER, and silent EMG is recognized with 46.9% WER. On the EMG-PIT pilot corpus, audible EMG is recognized with 37.9% WER, whereas for silent EMG, only 79.2% WER are attained.

There is a great variance between speakers: On the EMG-PIT pilot corpus we observe a few speakers where the recognition of silent EMG is relatively good, in particular, speaker 5, however for many other speakers, the cross-mode WERs are very high. The same observation is made on the EMG-UKA corpus: As for whispered speech, speakers 2 and 8 perform best both on the single-mode Sil → Sil setup and on the cross-mode setups, attaining silent speech Word Error Rates 30.5% and 31.5%, respectively. The other speakers perform worse. However, the results of each speaker are quite consistent (the standard deviation is low), which is a notable result: Since all speakers achieve good results on audible EMG, it is clear that the decline in recognition accuracy is due to the discrepancy between the audible and silent speaking modes.

6.3.2 Multi-Mode Training

In the second step, multi-mode systems using audible and silent speech are trained. As in section 6.2.2, we can train these systems on 80 training sentences, twice as much as the 40 training sentences with which the single-mode systems are trained. For comparison, we report results on multi-mode systems with 40 training sentences as well.

Figure 6.5 displays the results of this experiment, which are very similar across the two corpora: The WER of the 40-sentence multi-mode system is lower than the WER of the cross-mode systems, but higher than the WER of any of the single-mode systems, both on audible and silent EMG and on both corpora. Encouragingly, for 80 training sentences, we obtain a substantial improvement, and

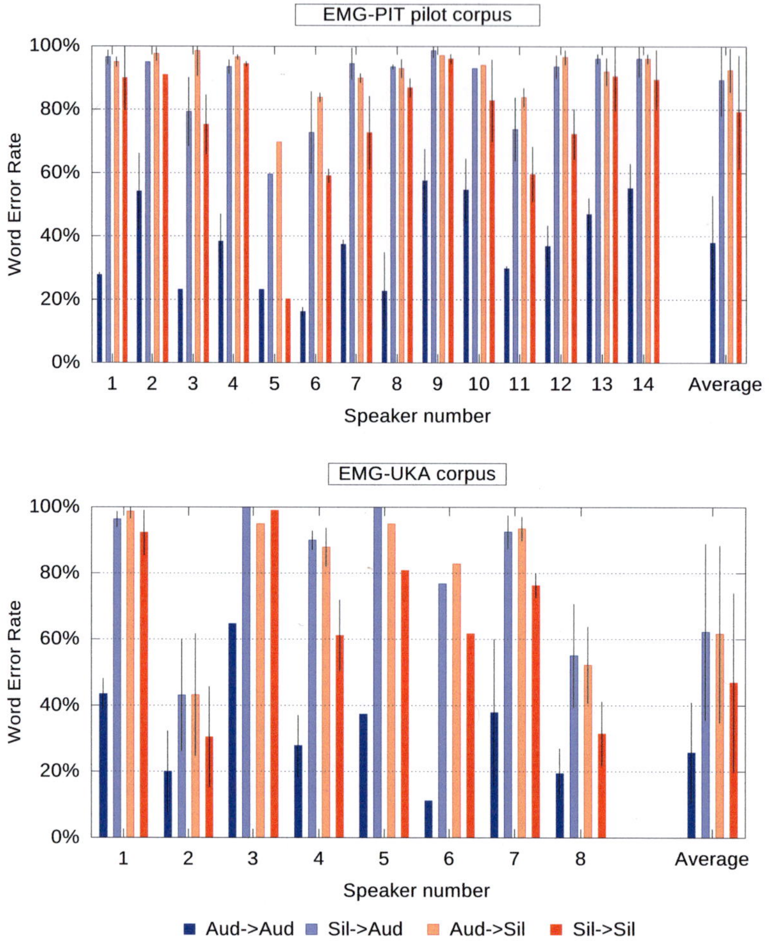

Figure 6.4 – Speaker breakdown of Word Error Rates for audible and silent speech. The label A $\rightarrow$ B means that the recognizer was trained on speaking mode A and tested on speaking mode B. Bars indicate standard deviation over sessions.

in particular, the 80-sentence multi-mode systems achieve clearly better recognition of *silent* EMG than the 40-sentence single-mode systems.

On *audible* EMG, the average WER is slightly higher for the 80-sentence multi-mode system than for the single-mode system. This is markedly different from the results on whispered EMG presented in figure 6.3, where we observed that

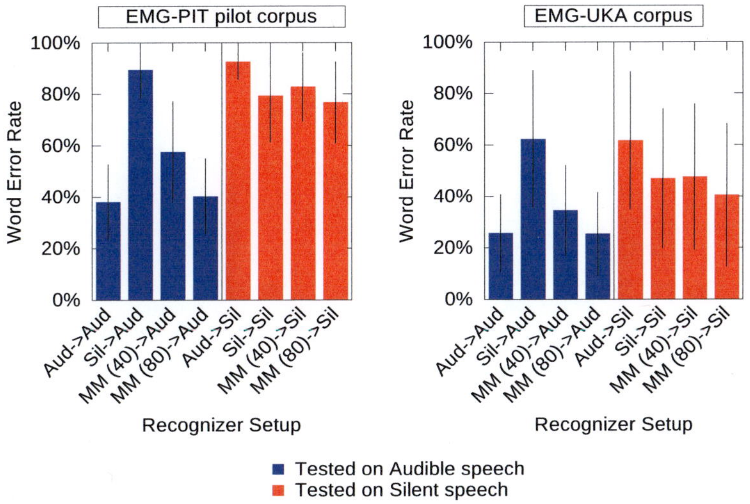

Figure 6.5 – Word Error Rates on audible and silent speech, for single-mode, cross-mode, and multi-mode (MM) training. The number in parentheses stands for the number of training sentences on the multi-mode systems. Bars indicate standard deviation.

both speaking modes profited from using 80-sentence multi-mode training; it must be concluded that the discrepancy between audible and silent EMG is far larger than between audible and whispered EMG.

As a final experiment in multi-mode training, we use the EMG-UKA corpus to train systems using the training sets from *all three* speaking modes. This means that 120 training sentences are used for each session. In figure 6.6, we compare the results on this setup to the results on different systems, namely on the single-mode recognizers, and additionally on the 80-sentence multi-mode recognizers trained on audible and silent resp. audible and whispered EMG.

We observe that applying the multi-mode system yields a WER improvement on all three speaking modes, yielding the best multi-mode WERs so far: audible, whispered, and silent EMG are recognized with 19.9%, 21.9%, and 38.4% WER, respectively. Altogether, we conclude that training multi-mode systems is feasible and yields good recognition rates. It should be noted that the results reported above do *not* depend on prior information about the speaking mode of the test data, so it should even be possible to switch the speaking mode in the middle of a sentence, e.g. to convey confidential information like PINs or passwords.

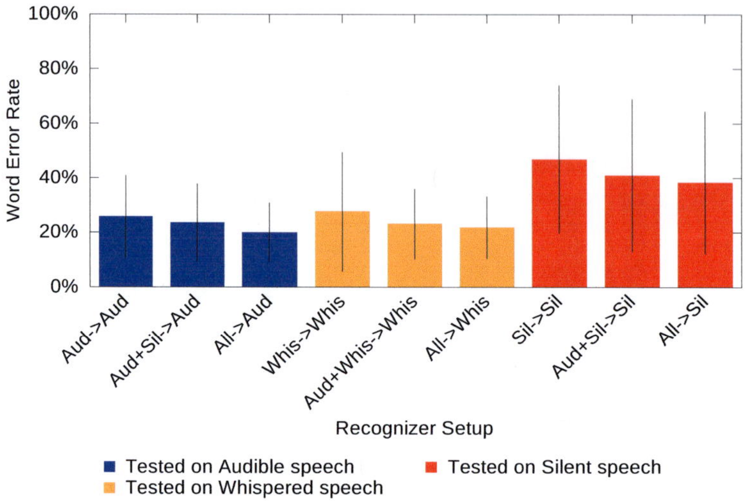

Figure 6.6 – Word Error Rates on audible, whispered, and silent speech, for different training setups (*all* stands for multi-mode training on all three speaking modes). Only the EMG-UKA corpus was used. Bars indicate standard deviation.

6.4 Quantification of Speaking Mode Variation by Phonetic Decision Trees

In this section we turn to developing measures to quantify the impact of speaking mode variabilities on the EMG-based speech recognizer. Unless stated otherwise, the results refer to the audible and silent speaking modes, since for the purpose of the EMG-based speech recognition system, silent speech is considered to be more important than whispered speech.

In order to evaluate the measures presented below, an estimate for the discrepancy between the audible and silent EMG data in a particular session is required. For this purpose we train a multi-mode recognizer on audible EMG and silent EMG and test it separately on the test sets of these two speaking modes. We then use the difference between the Word Error Rates between these speaking modes as a measure for their discrepancy.

Since good recognition of silent EMG is our primary goal, we assert that the *WER difference* is suitable for our purpose: it reflects the loss of accuracy when switching from audible to silent EMG test data. Note that the WER difference measure is session-dependent, just like our recognizers, so the variations in base-

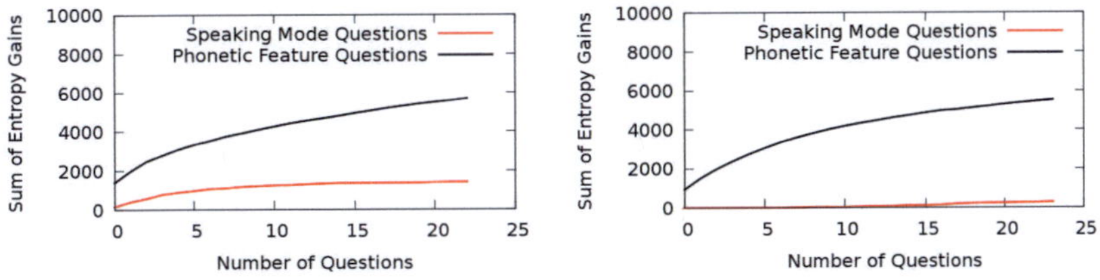

Figure 6.7 – Entropy gains for a speaker with high discrepancy (left)/low discrepancy (right) between the recognition performance on audible and silent EMG, plotted over the number of splitting questions asked. The results are averaged over all PF trees. The scaling of the vertical axis is arbitrary, it stems from the phonetic decision tree splitting algorithm.

line accuracy of different sessions which are not related to the speaking mode are factored out.

Obviously, the WER difference is an empirical measure which requires to train and apply the recognition system. Our first goal is to predict the speaking mode discrepancy, measured by the WER difference, ideally *without* having to train and test the recognizer, and without having to use the test data transcriptions as an oracle.

The method presented in this section considers the *phonetic decision trees* which the phonetic feature bundling algorithm uses to create optimal phonetic feature models, see section 5.2.2. This means that generating models, i.e. training the recognizer, is required, but no testing phase is needed in order to obtain a result. We first presented this approach in [WJS12], using an idea from [SW01].

The technique works as follows: We tag each phone of the training data set with its speaking mode (audible or silent). We then let the decision tree splitting algorithm ask questions about these attributes, in addition to the standard questions about phonetic features. When a model split is performed according to a speaking mode question, this indicates a discrepancy between audible and silent speech for the phonetic features and contexts collected in this model. The magnitude of this discrepancy is reflected in the entropy gain (see section 2.3.4) associated to this split. It should be noted that using speaking mode questions only has a minimal and inconsistent impact ($\pm$ 2%) on the average recognition results, so we do not separately report results on multi-mode systems with or without speaking mode questions.

We follow the approach from [SW01] and examine the *entropy gains* associated with the model splitting process: Figure 6.7 plots the cumulative entropy gain for speaking mode questions and phonetic feature questions over the total number of questions asked, for a speaker where the WER difference between audible and silent EMG speech is relatively large (left) respectively relatively small (right). The values are averaged over all eight PF trees. It can be seen that for the speaker with small WER difference, the speaking mode questions do not contribute much to the entropy gain at all, while in the case of a speaker with high WER difference, the speaking mode questions are responsible for a large amount of the entropy gain. Note that we limited the range of the horizontal axes of figure 6.7 to the total size of the smallest BDPF tree in the system.

This observation suggests to use the entropy gain as a discrepancy measure between audible and silent EMG. This approach draws its validity from the fact that BDPF bundling splits Gaussian mixture models in a *data-driven* manner without resorting to any kind of prior knowledge or assumption: thus the results of the algorithm give an insight into properties of the underlying models.

In order to obtain a single value describing the entropy gain, we consider all PF trees and look at the question which yields the *highest* entropy gain of all questions about the speaking mode. It is possible to use different criteria (e.g. averages over all speaking mode questions), but since in a decision tree questions are strictly sorted according to decreasing entropy gain, using the highest entropy gain has the advantage that this measure depends only on the first few questions of the decision tree.

We use this *maximum entropy gain* (MEG) as a measure for the discrepancy between speaking modes: If there is hardly any difference between speaking modes, the MEG should be small, possibly even zero if no speaking mode question at all has been asked. If the EMG signals of different speaking modes differ a lot, there should exist a high entropy gain associated to a speaking mode question. Note that it is entirely possible that a tree only contains one single speaking mode question (e.g. the very first question) which nonetheless yields the highest gain among all questions.

Figure 6.8 plots the MEGs for all the sessions of the EMG-UKA corpus (on the vertical axis) and compares them with the difference of the Word Error Rates of silent and audible EMG on the respective multi-mode system.

The maximum entropy gain varies across sessions from 0 to 1497, with an average of 441, and correlates with the WER difference between audible and silent EMG with a correlation coefficient of 0.70. The best session, where no questions about the speaking mode occur, is from speaker 2, the session with the highest entropy gain is from speaker 1. This shows that the MEG can, to a certain extent, predict the loss of recognition accuracy when switching between audible and silent speech. A more detailed analysis of figure 6.8 shows that there is a sizeable cluster of sessions with very low entropy gain and very low WER

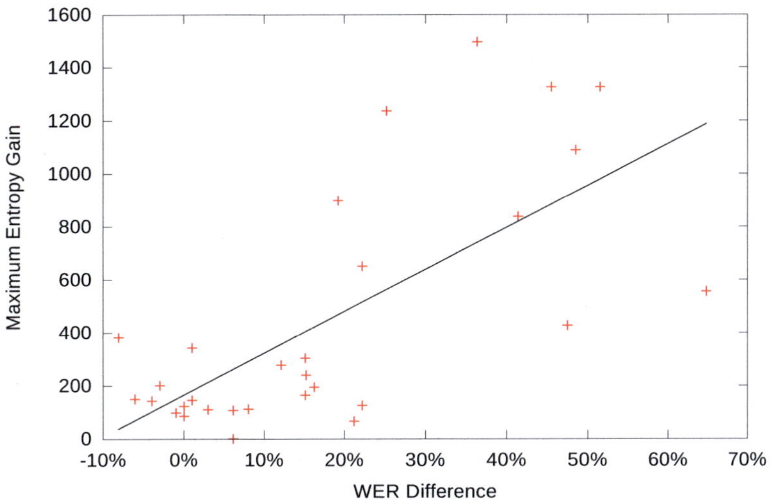

Figure 6.8 – Scatter plot of the Maximum Entropy Gain (MEG) and the WER difference per session between silent and audible EMG for the EMG-UKA corpus, with regression line.

difference, when the WER difference gets higher, we observe higher maximum entropy gains as well as a greater variation between different sessions.

For the EMG-PIT pilot corpus, we obtain a very different result: Here the MEG hardly correlates at all with the WER difference between silent and audible speech. In particular, for the second session of speaker 1, the MEG is zero, but the WER difference is 61%, i.e. silent EMG is recognized *far* worse than audible EMG. A closer inspection of the training process shows that in this session, the Viterbi algorithm, which computes the alignment of the EMG data as one step of the HMM training algorithm (see section 2.3.5 for a detailed description), failed to converge for almost all of the silent EMG utterances, so that no time-alignments are produced. In these cases, our training implementation automatically skips these utterances, so that eventually, almost no silent EMG training data is considered in this session. If the training data consists of mostly one speaking mode, speaking mode questions do not yield any gain and therefore do not occur, which explains the failure of the maximum entropy gain measure in this case.

This effect occurs with several other sessions of the EMG-PIT corpus as well, albeit not as extremely. Our attempts to modify the Viterbi algorithm by increasing the *beam* thresholds responsible for limiting the search space during the path calculation proved unsuccessful: This makes it clear that for some of the speakers in the EMG-PIT corpus, the quality of the silent EMG data is very bad, and it is also obvious that the entropy gain measure is not suitable for *very* large discrepancies between audible and silent EMG: At least, the model training must run without errors. We also note that the incomplete training of some of the sessions of the EMG-PIT corpus adversely affects the recognition results on the EMG-PIT corpus displayed in figures 6.4 and 6.5.

We also computed the maximum entropy gain measure on multi-mode systems trained with audible and *whispered* EMG from the EMG-UKA corpus, which were described in section 6.2. Since the cross-mode systems using whispered and audible EMG work comparatively well, we expect a lower MEG than for silent and audible EMG. Indeed, in this case the average MEG is only 87 compared to 441 for silent and audible EMG. Also, in 17 out of the 30 sessions no speaking mode questions at all are asked, so that the MEG is zero. While this proves that audible and whispered speech go along well, the correlation between the MEG and the WER difference between audible and whispered EMG is only 0.35, lower than for audible and silent EMG.

We conclude this section by presenting another model-based measure for the discrepancy between speaking modes, which we introduced in [WJS11]: In the phonetic decision trees, the fraction of tree leaves dependent on the speaking mode is counted [SM10, EGJM95]. Here a leaf node of the phonetic decision tree is considered "mode-dependent" if any question which is asked when traversing the tree from its root to the leaf asks for a speaking mode. The fraction of "mode-dependent tree nodes" (MDN) out of the set of all nodes is then used as a measure for the speaking mode discrepancy.

Computing this measure on the multi-mode sessions of the EMG-UKA corpus yields a fraction of MDNs ranging from 0.2% to 94.9%, with an average of 36.3%. Again we can compute the correlation between this measure and the WER difference, which is 0.64, slightly lower than for the maximum entropy gain. A further advantage of the maximum entropy gain is its robustness towards different sizes of the phonetic decision tree, which was described above: Due to the design of the tree growing algorithm, the speaking mode question which yields the maximum entropy gain is always the *first* speaking mode question *ever* asked. Thus when the stopping criterion for the decision tree growth is varied within reasonable limits, the maximum entropy gain measure never changes, whereas of course, the fraction of mode-dependent nodes may vary with different phonetic decision tree sizes.

We finally remark that both decision-tree based methods yield quite similar results over all eight PF trees. This is an indicator both for the robustness of

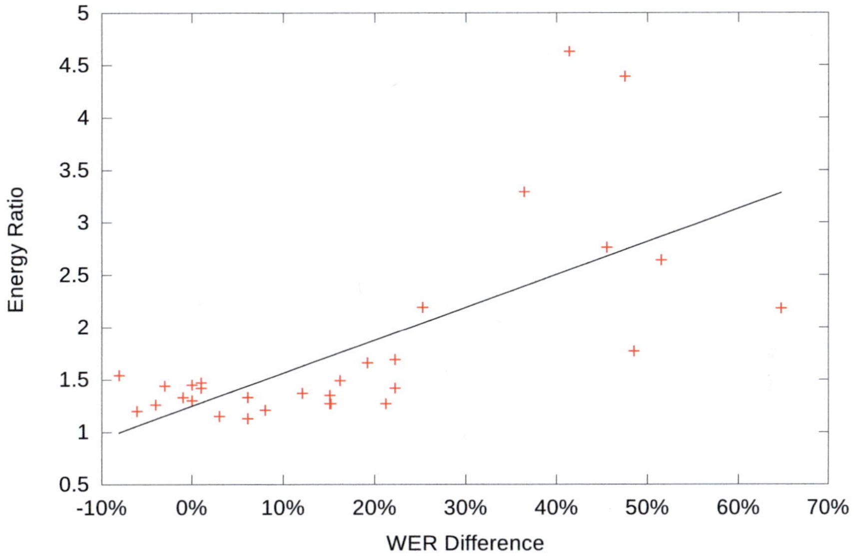

Figure 6.9 – Scatter plot comparing the average energy ratio of pairs of corresponding utterances and the difference of word error rates (WER) on silent and audible EMG for each session of the EMG-UKA corpus, with regression line. The WER difference is computed on the multi-mode system. The correlation coefficient is 0.69.

decision-tree based analysis of speaking mode discrepancies, and for the robustness of the BDPF models.

6.5 Energy-based Quantification of Speaking Mode Variations

In this section we turn to measuring the speaking mode discrepancy based on the EMG signals alone, without using the recognition system at all. A very simple measure is based on the *magnitude* of the EMG signals: In [WJTS09] we showed that the magnitude of the EMG signal of silent utterances is significantly lower than that of corresponding audible utterances, where *corresponding* utterances are defined as having the same textual content.

We can use this observation to define a speaking mode discrepancy measure based on the energies of the EMG signal [WJTS09]. We proceed as follows: For each EMG utterance, we compute the average energy by channel, defined by the formula

$$E = \frac{1}{N} \sum_{n=1}^{N} x_n^2,$$

where N is the number of samples, and $(x_n)_{n=1...N}$ is the raw EMG signal with normalized mean. Now we compute the *ratio* of energies for each pair of corresponding audible and silent EMG utterances, and finally, we average these ratios over all channels and all pairs of utterances.

Figure 6.9 displays a scatter plot of the energy ratio measure which was defined above versus the WER difference, computed on the EMG-UKA corpus. It can be seen that there is a relationship between the energy ratio and the WER difference, which behaves similar to the entropy gain: There is a cluster of sessions with small WER difference (up to 22%) and energy ratio close to one, whereas for sessions with high WER difference, the energy ratio is higher (1.7 and above). Remarkably, the energy ratio is *always* above one, which means that on average, we observe higher energy in audible EMG than in silent EMG in *all* sessions.

It can be seen from figure 6.9 that the majority of sessions exhibits reasonable difference between the recognition rates on audible and silent EMG, as well as relatively small energy ratios. The high correlation coefficient between the WER difference and the energy ratio is mainly due to a few "outliers", i.e. sessions with very high WER differences. Thus it must be concluded that predicting the value of the WER difference from the energy ratio may not yield optimal results in a practical setting. However, a coarser prediction with practical importance is possible.

We observe two groups of sessions, namely those with high WER difference (above 22%), and those with low WER difference. This boundary is of course not canonical (it is taken based on the observation in figure 6.9), but we consider it legitimate nonetheless, in particular since the low-WER sessions form a very compact group. Clearly, we desire to avoid obtaining sessions belonging to the first group.

Figure 6.9 shows that the category of a given session can be deduced from the energy ratio: All sessions with a WER difference above 22% also have energy ratios of above 1.7. Such a heuristical classification is helpful in practical scenarios: For example, if a speaker records audible and silent speech in order to prepare for using a multi-mode recognizer, the recording system could determine the energy ratio, which is possible in real time, and warn the speaker that the recorded data may be suboptimal if the energy ratio gets too high.

We also computed the energy ratio on the EMG-PIT pilot corpus. However we did not achieve robust results, which must probably be attributed to the low-

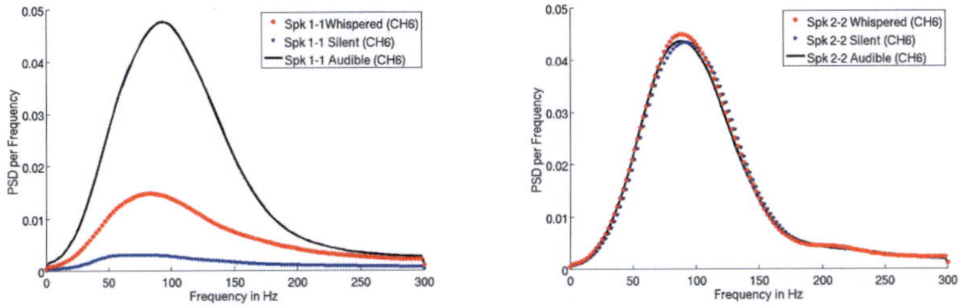

Figure 6.10 – PSD of EMG channel 6 of a silent speaker with high WER for cross-mode recognition (left) and a silent speaker with low WER across speaking modes (right). In the first case, the magnitude of PSD curves differs greatly, in the second case, almost no difference is observed.

frequency artifacts which are found in the EMG data of the EMG-PIT corpus, see section 3.1.1. While it should be possible in principle to filter out these artifacts, we refrained from doing so since the newer EMG-UKA corpus was recorded with an improved amplifier whose analog filter automatically took care of this issue.

6.6 Spectrum-based Quantification of Speaking Mode Variations

In [JWS10a, JWS10b], we presented another approach to measure speaking mode discrepancies, which extends and improves the energy-based method presented in the last section. In this approach we consider the energy content of the EMG signal *per frequency region* for audible, whispered, and silent EMG.

The method works as follows. First a spectral representation of the EMG recordings of one session is computed on a per-utterance and per-channel basis. In order to obtain a smooth estimate of the EMG spectrum, we base this computation on the *Power Spectral Density (PSD)*, which is a useful estimator for the smoothed frequency components of the EMG signals [JWS10a]. The PSD is estimated using *Welch's method* [Wel67]: The EMG signal is divided into windows with a length of 30 samples and an overlap of 20 samples, the FFT is computed on these windows, and the resulting spectra are averaged. Finally, the PSDs are averaged over all utterances.

As an example, the left part of figure 6.10 shows PSD curves of EMG channel 6 for the first session of Speaker 1. This speaker exhibits consistently high WERs on silent speech and on cross-mode recognition for whispered speech (see 6.4 and

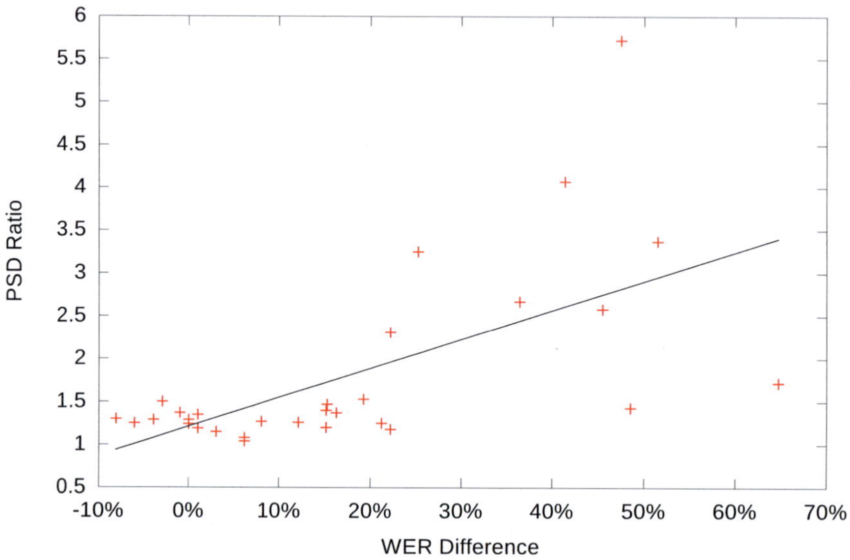

Figure 6.11 – Scatter plot comparing the ratio between power spectral density (PSD) of audible EMG and PSD of silent EMG and the difference of word error rates (WER) on silent and audible EMG for each session of the EMG-UKA corpus, with regression line. The PSD is maximized over frequency bins and averaged over all channels of a session, the WER for silent EMG is from the multi-mode system. See text for details.

6.2). The curve shapes are similar across modes, but the amplitudes differ for the speaking modes: In particular, the PSD of silent EMG is always much lower than the PSD of audible EMG. Whispered EMG is located in-between. The right part of figure 6.10 charts PSD curves of a well practiced silent speaker with good recognition rates for all speaking modes in all setups (single-mode, cross-mode, multi-mode). In this case, the PSD curves for audible, whispered, and silent EMG are almost identical.

This suggests that the spectral contents of the EMG signals may be used as a measure of the EMG signal discrepancy between speaking modes. In order to obtain a scalar value, we consider, for each EMG channel, the *ratio* between the PSDs of the audible EMG signal and the silent or whispered EMG signal as a function of the frequency. As before, this ratio is averaged over the utterances of a session. We finally take the maximum of this ratio, average over all channels, and so obtain a single value per session mirroring the difference between audible and whispered or silent EMG. This value is named *PSD Ratio*. Since this is our main target, we only consider silent speech.

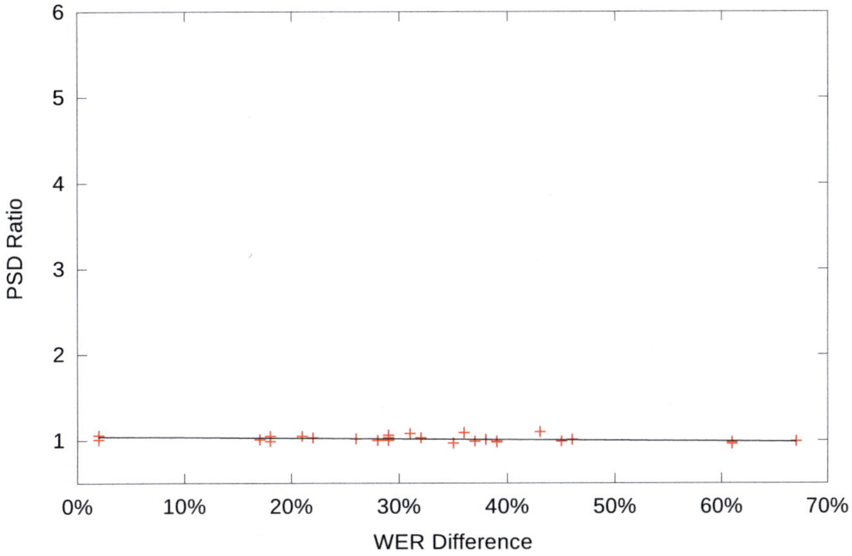

Figure 6.12 – Scatter plot comparing the ratio between power spectral density (PSD) of audible EMG and PSD of silent EMG and the difference of word error rates (WER) on silent and audible EMG for each session of the EMG-PIT pilot corpus, with regression line. The PSD is maximized over frequency bins and averaged over all channels of a session, the WER for silent EMG is from the multi-mode system. We observe that the results from the EMG-UKA corpus do not transfer. See text for details.

Figure 6.11 shows a scatter plot of the PSD ratio versus the WER difference between audible and silent speech, for each session of the EMG-UKA corpus. As for the Maximum Entropy Gain criterion (see figure 6.8), it can be observed that all sessions where the WER difference is low exhibit a small PSD ratio, whereas for sessions with higher WER difference, the PSD ratio may also increase. All PSD ratios are above one, i.e. for all sessions, the audible EMG spectrum contains more energy than the silent EMG spectrum on average. The WER difference is predicted quite well by the PSD ratio: the correlation coefficent is 0.63.

Similar to the energy ratio, the PSD ratio computation does not yield robust results on the EMG-PIT pilot corpus. Figure 6.12 shows a scatter plot of the PSD ratio versus the WER difference between audible and silent speech on the EMG-PIT pilot corpus: In stark contrast to figure 6.11, we see that for *all* speakers and sessions, without exception, the PSD ratio is very close to one. This clearly stems from the strong artifacts which are present in the EMG-PIT corpus (see section

3.1.1, in particular figure 3.4), and precludes using the PSD ratio to predict the performance of a speaker on silent speech: It is obvious that no relation between PSD ratio and WER difference can be derived from the data plotted in figure 6.12.

6.7 Spectral Mapping to Compensate Speaking Mode Discrepancies

So far, we have been *describing* the discrepancy between audible and silent speech. The spectrum-based approach described in the previous section allows even more: We can improve the recognition of silent speech with a frequency-based adaptation technique. This algorithm is called *Spectral Mapping*, we introduced it in [JWS10a]. It works as follows:

1. The utterances of a session are transformed into the frequency domain via the (fast) Fourier Transformation (FFT).
2. For each pair of parallel silent and audible EMG utterances, the ratio of the frequency components is computed. The result is averaged over all utterances of the session. We call this frequency-dependent ratio *mapping factor*.
3. Each silent EMG utterance is transformed into the frequency domain by the FFT, then each frequency component is multiplied by the corresponding mapping factor, and the resulting frequency representation of the signal is transformed back into the time domain by the inverse FFT. Note that audible EMG utterances are left unchanged.
4. After this procedure, features are extracted from the transformed signals as usual. The resulting features are then used for any of the training and testing approaches described in section 6.3.

We evaluate the Spectral Mapping algorithm on both the single-mode and the multi-mode recognizers, considering audible and silent EMG. Figure 6.13 shows the Word Error Rates for these systems, averaged over all sessions of the EMG-PIT pilot corpus and the EMG-UKA corpus.

The Aud→Aud system is not influenced by Spectral Mapping. The WER for the Sil→Sil system changes minimally, which is expected since training and test data are identically transformed: this suggests that our algorithm does not significantly distort the EMG signal. For both cross-modal systems we observe a significant gain: On the EMG-UKA corpus, the Aud → Sil system improves from 61.6% WER to 54.8% WER, which is an improvement of 11.0% relative, and the Sil

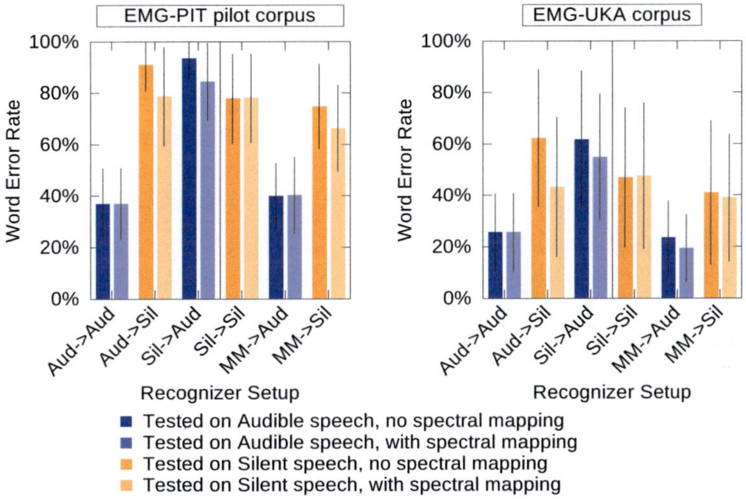

Figure 6.13 – Effect of Spectral Mapping. For each system, the left-hand bar shows the WER without Spectral Mapping, and the right-hand bar shows the WER with Spectral Mapping, where Spectral Mapping is always applied to the silent EMG training *and* test data. The label e.g. "Sil → Aud" indicates that the system was trained on the silent EMG training data and tested on the audible EMG test data. Bars indicate standard deviation.

→ Aud system improves from 62.2% WER to 43.3% WER, a substantial improvement of 30.4% relative. Similarly, we observe improvements on the EMG-PIT pilot corpus, although the absolute WERs are much higher: The Aud → Sil system improves from 93.4% WER to 84.4% WER (9.6% relative), and the Sil → Aud system improves from 90.9% WER to 78.7% WER (13.4% relative).

Substantial gains are observed on the multi-mode systems as well. On the EMG-UKA corpus, the WER of the multi-mode system on silent speech improves by 4.7% relative, on the EMG-PIT corpus, the improvement is 11.4% relative. When the multi-mode system is applied to audible EMG, the result is less clear: on the EMG-UKA corpus, we obtain an improvement of 17.8% relative, on the EMG-PIT corpus, no improvement is observed.

This shows that the Spectral Mapping algorithm helps to reduce the discrepancy between audible and silent EMG. This can also be observed by considering the Maximum Entropy Gain measure defined in section 6.4. When applying Spectral Mapping, we observe that for 29 out of 30 sessions, the maximum entropy gain decreases, the average of 441 reduces to only 182.

It is notable that Spectral Mapping also works on the EMG-PIT corpus, on which the PSD ratio discrepancy measure did not yield any consistent result. This is a strong indicator that the EMG-PIT data is not fundamentally different from the EMG-UKA data: instead, we consider it very probable that the artifacts contained in the EMG-PIT data negatively affect the PSD ratio, which is based on maximizing over all frequency bins, but do not preclude the application of Spectral Mapping, where all frequency bins are considered separately.

In our opinion, this also justifies that we refrained from improving our speaking mode discrepancy measures so that they would work on the EMG-PIT corpus: The newer EMG-UKA corpus does not contain these low-frequency artifacts, due to the improved amplifier which was used for the recordings, so this particular problem has been resolved. (Of course, there are definitely other kinds of artifacts in our corpora which are not suppressed by a high-pass filter. Also see section 7.4, which deals with artifact removal for the EMG-ARRAY corpus.)

As a final experiment, we applied Spectral Mapping to the multi-mode system trained on all three speaking modes. According to section 6.3.2, the average baseline WER without Spectral Mapping is 19.9%, 21.9%, and 38.4% on audible, whispered, and silent EMG, respectively.

We apply Spectral Mapping only to the silent EMG data, with the mapping factor being computed between silent and audible EMG, as described above. This yields a silent EMG WER of 34.8%, which is a relative improvement of 9.4%, i.e. the improvement is in the same range as for the other systems. The resulting WERs are 19.3% on audible EMG and 21.0% on whispered EMG, which is a slight improvement of 2.9% and 4.2% relative, respectively.

6.8 Statistical Evaluation

For statistical evaluation we use the main part of the EMG-PIT corpus, as usual. This means that we cannot validate any hypothesis including whispered EMG. Still, we have two hypotheses:

1. Spectral Mapping improves the silent EMG WER on a cross-mode recognizer trained on audible EMG
2. Spectral Mapping improves the silent EMG WER on a multi-mode recognizer trained on audible and silent EMG

The WER of the multi-mode system on *audible* EMG did not improve on the pilot part of the EMG-PIT corpus, and we expect this result to transfer to the main part. Therefore no hypothesis is made regarding that experiment.

System	Word Error Rate on Silent EMG		Improvement	
	no Spec. Map.	with Spec. Map.	relative	absolute
Cross-Mode	90.2%	79.8%	11.5%	10.4% ± 3.04%
Multi-Mode	80.2%	75.8%	5.5%	4.4% ± 1.95%

Table 6.2 – Word Error Rates of the cross-mode and multi-mode systems on silent EMG for the EMG-PIT main corpus

The resulting WERs and the absolute improvements with confidence intervals are displayed in table 6.2. For both systems we obtain significant improvements: The lower boundaries of the confidence intervals are well above zero. Thus we have established that the Spectral Mapping algorithm significantly improves the WER of our recongizer on silent EMG, even though the relative improvements somewhat vary on the different corpora. The best improvement is achieved on the evaluation corpus: The relative improvement of the cross-mode system is 11.5%.

6.9 Summary

In this chapter, we dealt with EMG-based speech recognition across different speaking modes. For this purpose, cross-mode and multi-mode recognizers were introduced. We showed that such recognizers work, although speaking mode discrepancies have a negative impact on their accuracies.

We analysed how such discrepancies manifest in the EMG data. This was done using measures at model level and at signal level. Our main observation was that signal energy discrepancies between audible and silent EMG correlate with the Word Error Rate difference between these speaking modes. Based on this observation, we devised the ***Spectral Mapping*** algorithm, a signal-based adaptation method specifically aimed at reducing the discrepancy between audible and silent EMG. We proved that Spectral Mapping significantly reduces the WER on silent EMG for both the cross-mode recognizer (trained on audible EMG) and the multi-mode recognizers, obtaining a maximum relative improvement of 11.5%.

Chapter 7

Array-based EMG Recording

In this section, we present a new EMG recording system based on ***Electrode Arrays****, which are grid structures with multiple measuring points for bioelectric signals. We report on initial experiments on deploying this new system and show that in contrast to our single-electrode systems, an additional PCA preprocessing step is necessary to obtain good baseline results. Finally, we introduce Independent Component Analysis (ICA) as a signal decomposition method and use it to define an artifact removal algorithm specially devised to take advantage of the high-dimensional EMG data which is obtained from electrode arrays.*

This chapter reports on our experiments using EMG signals recorded by *Electrode Arrays* [WSJS13]. Electrode Arrays are structures exhibiting a large number of electrodes arranged in a grid pattern, thus they yield a very comprehensive picture of the underlying EMG activity. However, this capability comes at a price: As is shown in this chapter, the resulting high-dimensional signal needs to be processed carefully in order to obtain a suitable feature representation and good speech classification accuracy.

One major goal of using EMG arrays is enabling the use of a large class of modern signal processing algorithms. These algorithms are specifically devised to make use of high-dimensional representations of an underlying signal to extract information which is not available if just one, or a few, channels are recorded. The most well-known examples for such algorithms are *(Blind) Source Separation* [Car98] and *Beamforming* [VB88]. Both aim at extracting activity sources from the input signal: in the case of Blind Source Separation, this is done making only weak statistical assumptions about the data, as described in section 7.4, for now it is our method of choice.

The high-dimensional input signal is expected to exhibit an obvious, but important property: its channels must contain information from *similar* sources, but recorded at *different* positions. This *spatial diversity* is the core of many signal decomposition algorithms, not only in biosignal processing. Intuitively, one could say that like studying an unknown physical object by looking at it from several directions, spatially diverse recordings can be used to analyze a complex signal from various "perspectives" in order to gain a better understanding.

A further advancement which we expect from the EMG array technology is to better localize activity. With the single-electrode system, each EMG channel contains a summation of signals from local activity sources, but there is no way to gain detailed information about what comprises this activity: EMG signals from different muscles and muscle fibers, as well as different kinds of artifacts, may have been captured. The situation is better when EMG arrays are used: In this case, source separation may be applied, and we showed that the extracted EMG sources can be localized within the area covered by the EMG array ([HJWS], see also [WHH+13]). Relatedly, when single electrodes are reattached between sessions, there is no way to algorithmically determine whether the exact same locations as before are recorded, or to compensate for a possible position shift. When EMG arrays are used, it is possible to compensate for an array repositioning by *interpolating* EMG signals between measuring points, and more importantly, it is possible to estimate the approximate position shift and rotation, as we show in [WSJS14]. Both these results are quite recent and cannot be covered in this thesis due to time constraints, yet we consider them an indicator of the potential of the EMG array approach.

The experiments presented here are based on the EMG-ARRAY data corpus, see sections 3.1.2 and 3.2.3. The remainder of this chapter is structured as follows: We first summarize current applications of electrode arrays, particularly from the EMG field. In section 7.2 we report on our baseline system, observing that the results exhibit some unexpected degradation, which we attribute to *under-training* during the LDA computation. Principal Component Analysis (PCA) is introduced in section 7.3 as a remedy for this problem, finally yielding our array-based baseline system; it is shown that this system exhibits similar performance as the ones trained on the single-electrode corpora. Starting from this system, in section 7.4 we present an artifact reduction algorithm using Independent Component Analysis (ICA) and show that it can yield improved Word Error Rates: This is the first concrete application of the electrode array technology.

7.1 Related Work in Electrode Array Technology and Application

Electrode arrays for EMG measurement were first applied in the 1980's for studies in the medical domain [MMS85, dLM88, RRS87]. Here, the primary concern is to break up the EMG signal into its constituent *Motor Unit Action Potential Trains (MUAPTs)* [LvDJ$^+$04, GOA05, HZ04, dLAW$^+$06], see section 2.1.2 for a detailed description of the emergence and properties of such MUAPTs.

MUAP decomposition algorithms detect single MUAPs in the time domain, which are then clustered into series. This clustering primarily considers the shape of the extracted action potentials, additionally a model of the time interval between discharges is used: The time between MUAPs stemming from the same motor unit is assumed to follow a Gaussian distribution, so the temporal distribution of these time intervals is a Gaussian process. This "background knowledge" yields information about the expected emergence of a particular MUAP within a series of MUAP discharges (i.e. a MUAPT), and is very important for decomposing superimposed activity sources[1].

MUAP clustering requires that extracted MUAPs may be compared for similarity. While the detailed implementation of this comparison varies between researchers, almost all methods draw their potential from the spatial diversity of the recorded signal, which is where EMG arrays come into play: Only by using the information from high-density multi-channel EMG recording, enough information for discriminating MUAPs is obtained. This sheds light on the core idea of electrode array recording, which we introduced above: EMG activity is recorded from slightly different "angles", i.e. locations, yielding different observations of essentially the same activity. From these observations, versatile algorithms allow to extract information which cannot be derived from a single-channel observation. However, it is important to craft an algorithm which makes use of these multiple observations. If EMG array data is used naïvely, without fusing information from different channels, no improvement over single-electrode systems should be expected.

Electrode arrays are not yet frequently used outside the medical and research communities, possibly because mobile, affordable, and easy-to-use amplification and recording devices are still under development. However, further practical applications have been considered, for example in prosthesis control

[1] This can be compared to speech recognition, where both an *acoustic model* and a *language model* are used (see section 2.3.6): The language model does not contain any information about the acoustic realization of words or utterances, but it yields indispensable background knowledge about the speech process.

[SG82, EHP01]. Here, the goal is to control a limb prothesis as intuitively as possible. EMG signals are a logical choice for this purpose (at least as long as muscular activity is still present), and since it is required to capture multiple control signals if a large number of degrees of freedom is desired (e.g. for controlling single fingers of a hand prosthesis), a small number of single electrodes may not yield sufficiently accurate information [CvdS09].

Finally, we remark that source localization for bioelectric signals has also been applied to electroencephalographic (EEG) signals; in fact, here the methods appear to be far more standardized than in the EMG field. As an example, we mention the *Low Resolution Brain Electromagnetic Tomography (LORETA)* method, which aims at detecting EEG activity sources and localizing them within the three-dimensional brain: This is a challenging problem since even a high-density EEG cap only offers a two-dimensional recording of EEG activity at the head surface. Yet, LORETA is an established procedure; for further reading, a classical review is [PMEKL02].

7.2 A Baseline System for High-Dimensional EMG-based Speech Recognition

In the first experiment (see our publication [WSJS13]), we use our BDPF recognizer, with optimal settings as determined in chapter 5, and feed it with the EMG features from the array recording system, which is described in detail in section 3.1.2. Here we made the observation that the amplitude of the raw EMG signals differs between the array setup and the single-electrode system, which may have an impact on the EMG features. For comparability, we chose not to vary the **TD**n features at this point, however we performed several initial experiments on feature extraction for the EMG-ARRAY corpus and found that it is advantageous to multiply the Zero-Crossing Rate feature (see section 4.1.2) with a renormalization factor of $1/100$, balancing for the smaller variance of the raw input EMG data. Also, in order to obtain more robust LDA estimates, we use LDA *regularization*, as described in section 2.4.3, with a regularization factor $\beta = 1.0$. We observed that this factor may be varied within a reasonable range without significantly changing the resulting WERs.

The first set of experiments is based on the development set of the EMG-ARRAY corpus, as laid out in section 3.2.3 (see table 3.4). We perform four different experiments, varying in the EMG array setup (16 or 35 channels) and in the amount of input data: As described in section 3.2.3, a subset of our sessions comprises 160 training sentences and 20 test sentences, so we can do (session-dependent)

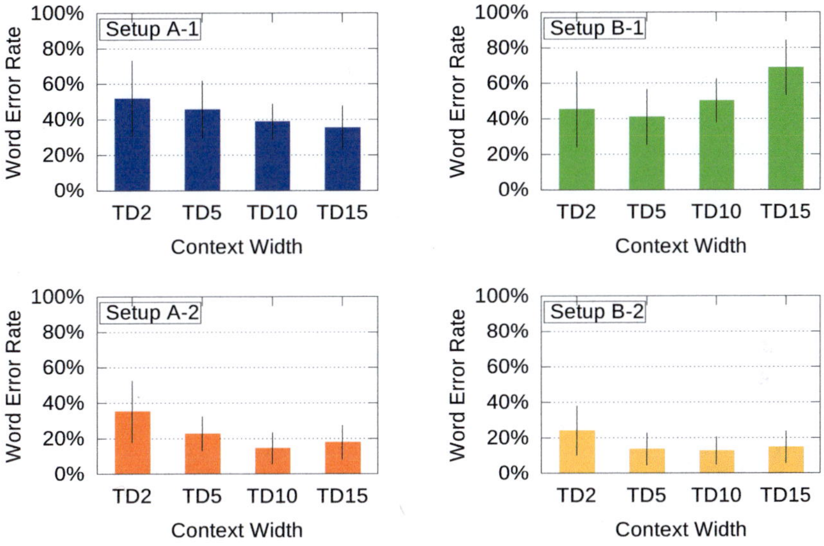

Figure 7.1 – Average Word Error Rates on the EMG-ARRAY development corpus for the initial array system, with different stacking context widths. Only audible EMG was used. Bars indicate standard deviation.

experiments on a substantially larger data set than in previous sections. In order to be able to compare our results to the ones from previous sections, we also run experiments with 40 training sentences and 10 test sentences. Only audible EMG is used.

Our four different setups are:

- *Setup A-1:* 16 EMG channels, 40 training sent., 10 test sent.
- *Setup A-2:* 16 EMG channels, 160 training sent., 20 test sent.
- *Setup B-1:* 35 EMG channels, 40 training sent., 10 test sent.
- *Setup B-2:* 35 EMG channels, 160 training sent., 20 test sent.

Figure 7.1 shows the Word Error Rates for different stacking widths, averaged over all sessions of each setup.

We consider the optimal context stacking widths for the four systems. One observes major differences: For setup A-1, with 16 channels and 40 training sentences, the Word Error Rate (WER) varies between 35.3% and 51.8%, with the optimum reached at a context width of 15 (i.e. **TD15**). For the B-1 setup, with 35 channels but the same amount of training data, the optimal context width appears to be **TD5** with a WER of 41.0%, widening the context causes deteriorating results, the worst WER is 68.7% for the **TD15** stacking.

For the setups with 160 training sentences, the recognition performance is consistently better due to the increased amount of training data. With respect to context widths, we observe that the A-2 setup, again with 16 EMG channels, attains its optimal performance at a stacking width of 10, with a WER of 14.6%, for setup B-2, **TD10** stacking is optimal, too, with a WER of 12.7%.

While the behavior of these systems varies between recording sessions (mostly due to the small test data set), there is a quite consistent trend which we observe over the four setups, namely, the optimal context width *decreases* when the number of input channels rises, and it *increases* when a larger amount of training data is available. The one exception is the A-2 setup. However, as shown in table 3.4, we have only three sessions for experiments with the A-2 setup, so we attribute this discrepancy to statistical inaccuracy. Notably, the trend gets more pronounced when a higher LDA dimensionality is used (as for example in [WSJS13], where we used 32 dimensions after LDA).

What might cause this behavior? It is clear that adding more context information might cause deteriorating results if the enlarged context is not consistent. This is certainly possible for our EMG data: The **TD15** feature stretches across more than 300 ms, a span which quite probably covers several adjacent phones. However, we see that a larger context is advantageous for the 16-channel systems, and that results should only gradually change when the stacking context width varies (see figure 4.6 for results on the single-electrode system). May context data have different properties in EMG data recorded with different setups?

A second hypothesis leads to the *Curse of Dimensionality* described in section 2.3: Increasing the feature vector dimensionality may cause deteriorating classification results if the system becomes *undertrained*, i.e. the models cannot be suitably estimated since the amount of training data is too small. This issue is evident in EMG-based speech recognition, as can be seen from our experiments in section 4.3: When the number of retained dimensions after the final LDA preprocessing step was increased beyond 12, the recognition accuracy decreased even though *more* information was fed into the system. However, the different setups A-1, A-2, B-1, and B-2 described above all use a post-LDA dimensionality of 12, so the GMM models should not be affected by the input data dimensionality.

We assume that the deterioration of recognition accuracy for small amounts of training data and high feature space dimensionalities is caused not by the GMM training, but by the LDA estimation itself. When an LDA transformation is computed with a small amount of training data relative to the sample dimensionality, the LDA within-scatter matrix becomes (almost) singular, as described in section 2.4.3. This has been observed to reduce the effectiveness of the LDA algorithm [QZH09] and quite probably is the case in our setup: With only a few minutes of training data, we may have a sample dimensionality before LDA of up to $35 \cdot 5 \cdot 31 = 5425$ for the 35-channel system with a **TD15** stacking.

7.3 PCA Preprocessing to Avoid LDA Sparsity

One established method to alleviate the numerical instability in high-dimensional LDA computation is an application of Principal Component Analysis (PCA) prior to LDA estimation [SW96]. Notably, PCA does not suffer from the same kind of numerical instability as LDA since its definition is not based on a maximization of a ratio (compare the LDA criterion (2.18) with the PCA criterion (2.11)). In this section we present our experiments on applying PCA prior to LDA to the task of EMG-based speech recognition using electrode arrays.

The algorithm is straightforward: We first compute **TD**n features as usual. Then, a dimensionality-reducing PCA transformation is estimated on the **TD**n features of the training data, and LDA estimation is subsequently run on the *transformed* training data. When both transformations have been computed, training and testing run as usual, with *all* data being transformed by both PCA and LDA.

The clear drawback of this method is that if *too many* PCA components are deleted, the resulting system performance should degrade since PCA ignores the data class assignments and could thus suppress information which is important for classification. So it is crucial to retain the right number of PCA components. One might automatically determine this number from the data, but as described in section 2.4.2, we have not yet applied such methods and therefore always fix the number of retained PCA components across all speakers and sessions.

Besides the introduction of PCA preprocessing, all other system parameters (in particular, the number of LDA components) are kept fixed, so that comparisons can be made and conclusions can be drawn. We evaluate our algorithm by running session-dependent training and testing, as usual, and expect to obtain an improved WER as long as the PCA parameters are suitably chosen. Beyond an improved recognition accuracy, we also expect a more consistent result regarding the optimal feature stacking width.

Figure 7.2 presents the average WERs for all four setups, with different numbers of components after the PCA step. The leftmost data point is the average WER for 100 retained components, from left to right, the number increases up to the entirety of available components. The result without PCA application is on the

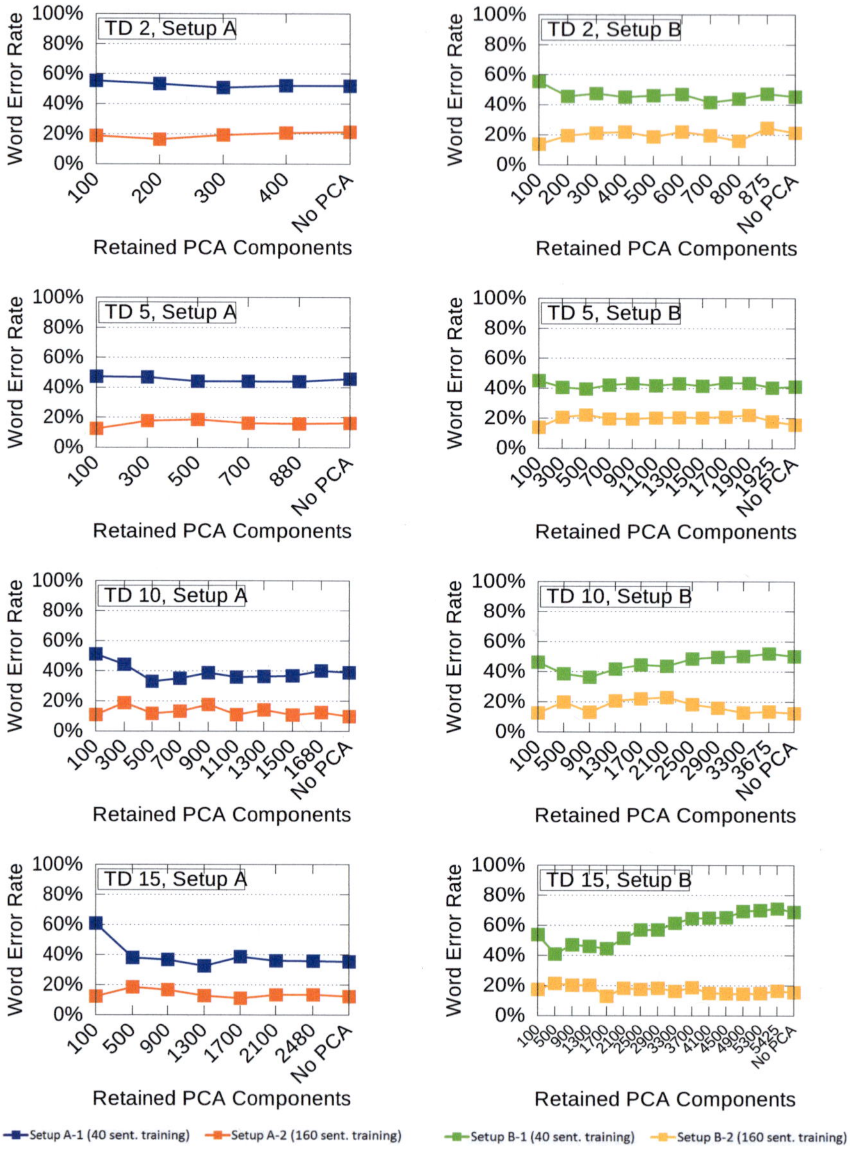

Figure 7.2 – Word Error Rates on the EMG-ARRAY development corpus for different PCA dimensionality reduction setups. Only audible EMG was used. Observe that the feature space dimension *before* the PCA step increases from left to right and from top to bottom.

Setup	A-1	A-2	B-1	B-2
Best Result without PCA	35.3%	14.6%	40.1%	12.7%
Opt. Stacking Width without PCA	15	10	5	10
Opt. Number of Dimensions without PCA	2480	1680	1925	3675
Best Result with PCA	32.5%	16.0%	36.2%	10.9%
Opt. Stacking Width with PCA	15	15	10	10
Opt. Number of Dimensions with PCA	1300	2100	900	1700
Relative Improvement by PCA	7.9%	-9.6%	11.5%	14.2%

Table 7.1 – Optimal Results and Parameters with and without PCA, on the EMG-ARRAY development corpus

very right. In all cases, we jointly plot the WERs for training data sets 1 and 2 (40 and 160 training sentences).

We see that the PCA step indeed helps to overcome LDA sparsity. For example, in the B-1 setup, the optimal context width without PCA application is 5, yielding a WER of 40.1% (right side, second plot from top). With PCA application, the optimal number of retained PCA dimensions for the **TD5** context width is 500, yielding a WER of 39.4%: a very slight improvement. However, we can still do better: With a substantially increased context width of 10, we get the best WER of 36.2%, at a dimensionality of 900 after PCA application (right side, third plot from top). This is an improvement of 11.5% relative.

This is true for three of the other four setups, see table 7.1 for an overview. For setup B with 35 EMG channels, we always obtain relative improvements of more than 10%, and for the B-1 setup, the optimal context width increases, as expected. For setup A with only 16 EMG channels, we obtain lower improvements: For 40 training sentences, i.e. setup A-1, the improvement is 7.9% relative, and for 160 training sentences, i.e. setup A-2, PCA brings no improvement. This is a consistent result: In the A-2 setup, the ratio between training data amount and data dimensionality is largest, so the LDA sparsity problem should be least pronounced here. We note that there is some variation in the optimal PCA dimensionality, which we do not consider to be statistically significant since for all setups we have relatively few sessions to experiment with; however we see that with only 100 retained PCA components, we frequently obtain very bad results: this is expected since with so many suppressed PCA components, we certainly suppress some relevant information as well. We also note that the effect of PCA increases when a higher LDA dimensionality is chosen: In [WSJS13], we report results of PCA application when 32 dimensions are retained after LDA, in that case, the improvements by PCA application exceed 10% relative in all four setups.

Setup	B-1		B-2	
Tested on	Aud. EMG	Sil. EMG	Aud. EMG	Sil. EMG
No Spectral Mapping				
WER without PCA	43.1%	71.2%	24.7%	62.6%
WER with PCA	41.0%	70.6%	24.6%	63.7%
With Spectral Mapping				
WER without PCA	44.4%	70.4%	25.0%	56.2%
WER with PCA	40.8%	67.9%	26.4%	56.2%

Table 7.2 – Results for multi-mode systems on the evaluation corpus. For the B-1 setup, we used **TD5** stacking without PCA, and **TD10** stacking with PCA (900 retained components). For the B-2 setup, we used **TD10** stacking without PCA, and **TD10** stacking with PCA (1700 retained components).

Finally, we perform statistical validation of our results on the evaluation part of the EMG-ARRAY corpus. Note that only setup B was recorded in the evaluation corpus since with optimal settings, our initial experiments showed that it yields better average WERs than setup A. We run two experiments, namely using setups B-1 and B-2, where the sets of sessions for the two experiments are identical: the entire B-1 data is a subset of the B-2 data. For now, we only use audible EMG.

Our hypothesis is that PCA preprocessing, with the optimal stacking width and optimal number of retained dimensions, yields an improvement over the best setup without PCA. The optimal settings are taken from table 7.1: The B-1 experiments use **TD5** stacking without PCA, and **TD10** stacking with PCA, where after the PCA application, 900 components are kept. For the B-2 experiments, we always use **TD10** stacking, when PCA is applied, 1700 components are kept.

On the B-1 setup, we obtain a WER of 47.4% without PCA, and 42.3% with PCA application. This is an *absolute* improvement of 5.1% with ± 3.0% confidence interval, so the improvement is statistically verified.

On the B-2 setup, we surprisingly do not obtain any improvement at all: Instead, the WER rises from 20.18% without PCA to 20.71% with PCA, which is insignificant, but nonetheless a degradation. We can explain the discrepancy between the two evaluation setups by the larger amount of training data for the B-2 setup (160 versus 40 training sentences). Still, it is clear that the effect of PCA application was overestimated on the four-session B-2 development corpus.

Finally, table 7.2 displays evaluation results on *multi-mode* systems trained on audible and silent EMG (see section 6.3). These systems use the full training data of the sessions of the EMG-ARRAY evaluation corpus, i.e. 80 sentences (40 audible and 40 silent) in case of the B-1 setup, and likewise, 320 sentences in case of the B-2 setup. Yet we keep the evaluation parameters fixed: For the B-1 setup, we compare **TD5** stacking without PCA and **TD10** stacking with PCA, using 900 PCA components. For the B-2 experiments, **TD10** stacking is used, with 1700 retained components when PCA is applied. We also display results both with and without Spectral Mapping, see section 6.7.

The result confirms our observations on audible EMG. On the B-1 setup, PCA application yields an improvement, the largest one of 8.1% relative is obtained on audible EMG test data when Spectral Mapping is applied. However, these improvements do not turn out to be significant. On the B-2 setup, we do not obtain improvements. We finally note that these experiments also support our result from section 6.7: Spectral Mapping improves the recognition accuracy of multi-mode systems on *Silent* EMG. In particular, we observe major improvements on the B-2 setup.

We finally remark that in [WSJS13], we reported results on this experiment with an LDA dimensionality of 32, which can be assumed to give more room for sparsity problems. Indeed, the reported improvements obtained by PCA application are substantially higher, particularly for setup A; see [WSJS13, Table 1].

We can draw the conclusion that at least for the 35-channel setups and for the given amount of training data, PCA preprocessing helps to overcome LDA sparsity. There remains the question whether this result is optimal, in the sense that the LDA sparsity problem is completely solved. The results in figure 7.2 suggest that the results could be even better: For example, we see that for the A-1 setup, **TD15** features yield good results. Even if this result does not transfer to the A-2 setup, we conclude that high context widths do carry information which help to classify speech based on EMG signals. Yet for setup B, we see that the results are worse for **TD15** features than for **TD10** features.

We conclude that even the PCA preprocessing does not completely solve the issue of optimal LDA computation. This means that very high-dimensional input data is still problematic, and that the context width must be chosen somewhat smaller for high-dimensional input data than for low-dimensional input data. We *can*, however, confirm a result from our baseline system, namely that the optimal context width when LDA sparsity is *not* an issue ranges between 10 to 15 frames on each side, as we determined in section 4.3. This may be derived from figure 7.2: For setup A, when PCA is applied with the optimal number of retained components, the resulting WER remains almost unchanged between the **TD10** and **TD15** features, for both 40 or 160 training sentences. This means that almost no additional information can be derived from the enlarged context. The observation is similar for the B-2 setup. Only for the B-1 setup, where the input

Corpus	Average WER
EMG-PIT (pilot)	34.0%
EMG-UKA	22.8%
EMG-ARRAY (setup A)	32.5%
EMG-ARRAY (setup B)	36.2%

Table 7.3 – Comparison of average Word Error Rates on audible EMG for the single-electrode corpora and the EMG-ARRAY corpus, with 40 training utterances

data dimensionality is highest and the number of training sentences is small, **TD15** performs worse than **TD10**, albeit just slightly when PCA is used.

One method to further improve the LDA estimation might be to determine the optimal number of PCA components on a per-session basis. However, this is expected to be time-consuming if the measure should be the resulting recognition accuracy: then repeated recognition runs would have to be performed on a cross-validation set. There also exist other, advanced LDA estimation methods (for example HLDA [KA98]), which have been used successfully in acoustic speech recognition and other fields.

In the remainder of this section, we use PCA+LDA (with optimal settings) as our new standard preprocessing for the EMG-based speech recognition system. Thus we now have three "baseline" results, namely, on the EMG-PIT (pilot) corpus, on the EMG-UKA corpus, and on the two setups A and B of the EMG-ARRAY corpus, always using 40 training sentences and 10 test sentences. Table 7.3 summarizes the average WERs and shows that the EMG-ARRAY corpus performs reasonably well.

7.4 Independent Component Analysis for Artifact Removal

We now present an artifact removal algorithm based on the multi-channel EMG signal provided by electrode arrays. This algorithm, which we published in [WHH$^+$13, WJH$^+$ar], is the first application of the newly introduced array-based recording setup: Beyond yielding recognition accuracy improvements, it shows that EMG-based speech recognition can be improved by using information contained in high-dimensional EMG signals. We first give an introduction into the concept of source separation and independent component analysis, upon which our method is based, then we present and evaluate our algorithm.

7.4.1 Review of Blind Source Separation and Independent Component Analysis

Quoting the comprehensive reference paper [Car98], *Blind Signal Separation (BSS)* "consists in recovering unobserved signals or 'sources' from several observed mixtures". The key assumptions which are expressed in this statement is that we have an underlying superposition of activity sources, that only mixtures of these sources can be observed (measured), *and* that we have several measurements.

We give a very brief overview about the principles of source separation, which lead to Independent Component Analysis (ICA) as a particular approach. The following exposition is based mostly on [Car98], for background on information-theoretic measures we refer to textbooks like [CT91].

First we define the term *mixture.* So assume that we have M signal sources $s_1, \ldots, s_M$, where each s_m is a digital signal: $s_m = (s_m[0], s_m[1], \ldots, s_m[N])$. Now the most general set of mixtures x_k, $k = 1, \ldots, K$ which one could possibly observe consists of the input signals, processed as a whole by arbitrary functions Φ_k:

$$x_k = \Phi_k(s_1, \ldots, s_M) \quad \text{with} \quad x_k = (x_k[0], x_k[1], \ldots).$$

Note that there is no reason to assume that the Φ_k acts on each sample independently: Instead, each Φ_k might transform all input sequences as a whole. Also note that K needs not equal M.

What constraints do we have to impose on Φ in order to have a reasonable chance of estimating the source sequences s_m? For the purposes of this introduction, we first assume *linearity*: Each source sequence undergoes a linear transformation, and each mixture consists of a summation of the transformed sources. The assumption of linearity is approximately satisfied in many practical applications (for example, air waves exhibit linearity properties), but might also be inaccurate (e.g. glass fiber cables might allow nonlinearly propagating waves). If we additionally assume that the properties of the transformation do not change over time, the mixing function may be expressed by linear *filters*:

$$x_k = \sum_{m=1}^{M} f_{k,m} * s_m, \tag{7.1}$$

where the $f_{k,m}$ are filters, and $*$ represents the convolution operation. Filters are a very important concept in signal processing and frequently occur in nature, a particular example which is of relevance for us is the vocal tract filter, see section 2.2.1. For more information about filters, we refer to standard signal processing textbooks (e.g. [KK02], in German language).

Convolutive mixtures, as in equation (7.1), can be inverted if some assumptions are satisfied. The approach is then called *(Blind) Deconvolution*, and several solutions have been proposed, see for example [BS95, AS98]. For "classical" Independent Component Analysis, we make an even stronger assumption, namely that the mixture is *instantaneous*:

$$x_k[n] = \sum_{m=1}^{M} a_{k,m} s_m[n] \quad \text{for any time } n. \tag{7.2}$$

Each sample $x[n]$ depends only on the sources at time n. This is the "textbook" source separation task, and several well-established algorithms may be used to find a solution. Yet depending on the concrete task, the assumption of instantaneousness may be too strong, and it means that we disregard the temporal evolution of the sources, even though it could be helpful for solving the source separation problem.

We are now able to define the classical Blind Source Separation task. First, we write equation (7.2) in matrix form, obtaining

$$x = A \cdot s \tag{7.3}$$

where $x = (x_1, \ldots, x_K)^T$ and $s = (s_1, \ldots, s_M)^T$ are vectors of time series. The goal is to invert the mixture. This essentially means inverting the matrix A, which is only possible if it is quadratic: Thus we make the additional assumption that there are as many sources as there are mixtures. For real-world signals, this is certainly a doubtful assumption, since sometimes the number of sources is not even known: It might be more accurate to say that we expect to extract exactly as many components as there are observed mixtures.

It should be clear that even the simplified matrix equation (7.3) cannot be solved without further assumptions, because neither A nor s are known. So we have to make an additional assumption, which is the cornerstone of classical BSS, namely, the sources $s_1, \ldots, s_M$ are assumed to be *statistically independent.* In terms of probability distributions, this can be expressed as follows: If s_i follows a probability distribution $p_i(\varsigma_i)$, written $s_i \sim p_i$, and the vector s has the M-dimensional distribution $p(\varsigma_1, \ldots, \varsigma_M)$, i.e. $s \sim p$, then p can be decomposed as

$$p(\varsigma_1, \ldots, \varsigma_M) = \prod_{m=1}^{M} p_m(\varsigma_m).$$

The independence condition is a constraint both strong and weak: It is a mathematically strong condition on the joint distribution of the sources, yet it does not restrict the behavior of the single sources at all. There is the notable result that this assumption *almost* suffices to determine an inverse of A from equation (7.3). The last missing piece is to require that out of the signal sources we intend to recover, *at most one* has a Gaussian distribution. Then one can show the following theorem (cp. [Com94, Theorem 11]):

Assume that $x = A \cdot s$, where A is an invertible (square) matrix, and s is a vector of independent "sources", of which not more than one follows a Gaussian distribution. If the matrix B is chosen so that the components of $y = B \cdot x$ are independent, then the vector y contains the sources s, up to reordering and rescaling.

This means that if we manage to find an *unmixing matrix* B which makes the components of $y = B \cdot x$ independent, the BSS problem is solved. Further knowledge of the sources is not required, which explains the naming "*Blind* Source Separation".

B is uniquely determined up to reordering or rescaling of its rows. Clearly, this is the best solution one can obtain, since there is no way to determine the original order of the s_m from the mixtures (in real-world applications, there is, of course, no "original order"), and the original scaling of the sources is equally lost by the mixing. Clearly, the assumption that the signal sources must be independent and non-Gaussian might be inaccurate for certain problems.

There are several ways to determine B, and we note that they differ in practice more than in theory: If the conditions are optimal, the solution B should be the same in all cases. Yet in practice, particularly if the amount of observed data for estimating B is small, different BSS algorithms may vary in performance.

First, there are BSS approaches which are based on the existence of a model assumption for the true distribution of the source vector s. If such a model exists, one can optimize B so that the distributions of y and s match as closely as possible. The discrepancy between the distributions of y and s can be measured by the *Kullback-Leibler divergence*, which is easily computed. Clearly, with such an approach we step back from the true idea of *Blind* Source Separation, however it can be (empirically) shown that such algorithms are quite robust even if the model for the distribution is slightly misspecified, and it can be (theoretically) shown that the model assumption can be greatly weakened: instead of computing the mismatch between distributions, it may be sufficient to compute the mismatch between higher-order statistical measures (e.g. cumulants). So instead of having a detailed model for the source distribution, it may be sufficient to have knowledge about some rather general properties of the sources (like the cumulants, or the higher-order moments).

Blind Source Separation approaches rely on approximations of the *mutual information*, which measures the degree of dependence between two random vari-

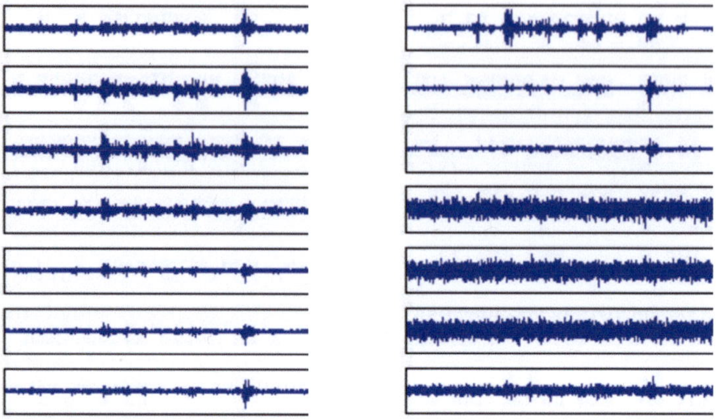

Figure 7.3 – EMG Signals of the chin array before ICA processing (left) and after ICA processing (right). The ICA decomposition shows visibly distinct EMG signal ("target") components (1 - 3) and artifact noise (4 - 7).

ables. If we have two random variables X and Y, defined by their density functions $p_X(x)$ and $p_Y(y)$ and the joint density $p(x,y)$, their Mutual Information is defined by

$$MI(X,Y) = \int p(x,y) \log \frac{p(x,y)}{p_X(x)p_Y(y)}.$$

x and y may be scalar variables or vectors.

It is easily shown that the mutual information is zero if X and Y are independent, and greater than zero otherwise. Thus for the BSS problem, one can use the mutual information between the components of the estimated source vector $y = B \cdot x$ as an optimization target, giving rise to *Independent Component Analysis*.

Unfortunately, estimating the mutual information from observed data is quite complicated, and it is even more complicated to estimate a gradient in order to update the matrix B. So the standard implementations of ICA always use an approximation of the mutual information, often based on cumulants. For our experiments we use the Infomax ICA algorithm according to [BS95], as implemented in the Matlab EEGLAB toolbox [DM04], and we refer to [BS95] for details about the implementation of the optimization.

7.4.2 The Artifact Detection and Removal Algorithm

Before proceeding to the description of the artifact removal algorithm, it is instructive to visually inspect the results of the ICA decomposition of our EMG signals. One typical example is shown in figure 7.3, where one sees a short part of a recording (chin array in bipolar configuration) on the left side, and the ICA decomposition on the right side. The decomposition matrix was estimated on the data from an entire session, and we note at this point that we always apply ICA to the two arrays (chin and cheek) *separately*, since both arrays capture very different EMG sources.

We see in figure 7.3 (left part) that the original EMG channels look quite similar to each other. This is unsurprising, since these EMG signals were measured at very close points; the inter-electrode distance for the chin array is only 5mm. We also see that there is some amount of noise interference. We infer from the figure that considered by themselves, adjacent channels contain *almost* identical information, and if only naïve feature extraction is used, one could probably leave out several of the channels without experiencing recognition accuracy degradation.

There is substantially more information available than can be seen in the raw signals: The ICA decomposition (figure 7.3, right part) yields three components which appear to contain EMG, we call them *target components.* The other four ICA components appear to contain noise. We expect that the removal of the noise channels before feature extraction improves the recognition results. We developed two strategies, which we initially reported in [WHH$^+$13, Him13, WJH$^+$ar]:

- **Direct method**: As described above, we take the ICA components, identify and remove artifact components, and then compute the EMG features on the *remaining ICA components.*
- **Backprojection**: We take the ICA components, identify and remove artifact components as before, and then back-project these components to the original signal. Mathematically, this can be described as applying the ICA decomposition, setting the artifact ICA components to zero, and then multiplying the altered set of ICA components with the *inverse* of the ICA matrix. From the back-projected signals, we now compute EMG features as usual.

In addition, we can extract features from the ICA components without removing any artifact components, and we compare the resulting WER to the baseline system without ICA application.

Artifact components are identified by the following three measures, which are computed on the ICA components and which we initially described in

[WHH$^+$13]. The thresholds were tuned on the development part of the EMG-array corpus, a description on how the optimal thresholds were determined is found in [Him13].

- Autocorrelation measure: This method typically identifies very regular (periodic) artifacts, like power line noise. We compute the autocorrelation sequence of the ICA component and then take the value of the *first maximum* after the first zero-crossing of the sequence. This value is a measure for the degree of periodicity of the sequence. If it is greater than 0.5, this component is deemed an artifact.

- High-frequency noise detection: The surface EMG signal has frequency range of 0Hz - 500Hz [ZX11]. Therefore a component with distinct high-frequency parts is considered an artifact. We compute the discrete-time Fourier transform of the ICA component and divide the frequency axis into two intervals: The "signal" interval from 0Hz to 500Hz, and the "noise" interval from 500Hz to 1024Hz (the Nyquist frequency). We then compute the areas of the amplitude of the Fourier transform over the two intervals and divide the "signal" area by the "noise" area. If the quotient is smaller than 1.3, this component is deemed an artifact.

- EMG signal range: The main energy of the EMG signal is found between 50Hz and 150Hz [ZX11]. As before, we take the ICA component and divide the frequency axis into two parts: A "signal" interval from 50Hz to 150Hz, and "noise" part from 0Hz to 50Hz and from 150Hz to 1024Hz. Then we divide the "signal" area by the "noise" area. If the quotient is below 0.25, we deem this component an artifact. For this measure, we found that the power spectral density yielded slightly more robust estimates than a standard Fourier transformation.

Our measures are first computed on each ICA component of *each utterance* of the training data set. In a second step, we combine the results: For a component to be considered an artifact, we require that *at least one* of the three methods considers this component an artifact on *a minimum percentage* of (training) utterances. This "artifact threshold" is varied between 35% and 95%, where a lower value causes more components to be removed. We observed that the threshold makes a difference when components vary across utterances, e.g. when the contact between electrode and skin deteriorates over time; yet there are only few components which exhibit such behavior.

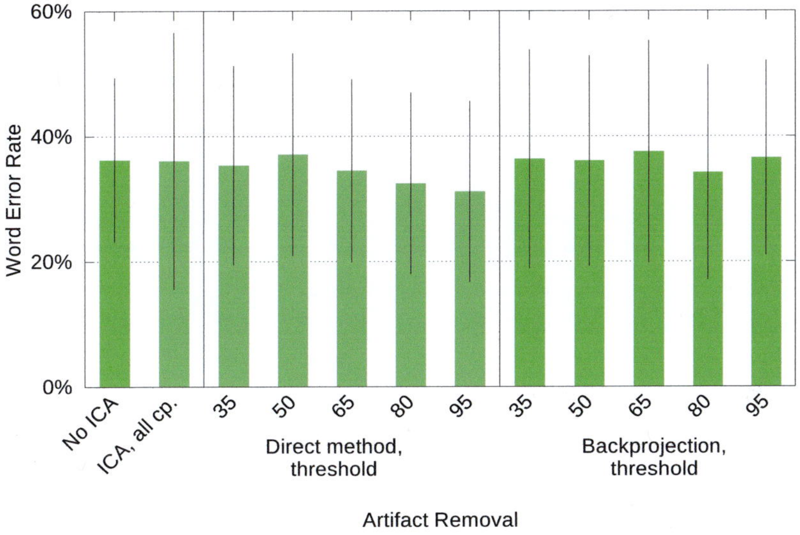

Figure 7.4 – Average Word Error Rates of the ICA-based artifact removal algorithm with different artifact thresholds on the development corpus, B-1 setup. Only audible EMG was used. Bars indicate standard deviation.

7.4.3 Evaluation of the Artifact Removal Algorithm

We evaluate the ICA-based artifact removal algorithm on the development set of the EMG-ARRAY corpus. Thus we have four setups, namely the setups A-1, A-2 (with 16 EMG channels) and B-1, B-2 (with 35 EMG channels). We also have different artifact removal configurations:

- No ICA application at all. The system computes features from the raw EMG data.
- The system uses ICA preprocessing, but *without* any artifact removal.
- *Direct method:* We compute the ICA decomposition of the signals, remove artifact channels as determined by our algorithm, and then compute EMG features from the remaining ICA components.
- *Backprojection*: We remove artifact components from the ICA data as before, and then process the remaining components with the inverse ICA matrix.

The latter two methods additionally allow the variation of the artifact threshold. In all cases, PCA+LDA is applied to the extracted features, with the exception

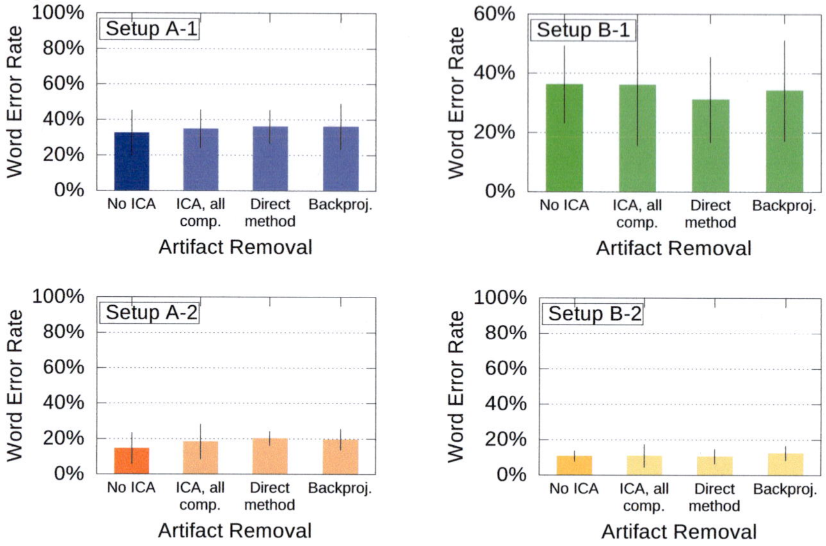

Figure 7.5 – Average Word Error Rates with the ICA-based artifact removal algorithm, for all four setups. Bars indicate standard deviation.

of the A-2 setup, where we use LDA but not PCA according to table 7.1. The optimal **TD**n stacking context width and the optimal number of retained PCA components are taken from table 7.1.

Results on all configurations for the B-1 setup are shown in figure 7.4. The optimal settings for the B-1 setup were used, namely TD10 stacking and PCA application with 900 components after the PCA step. One can see that in this case, ICA without artifact removal yields an insignificant improvement: The WER drops from 36.2% to 36.1%. If artifact components are removed, the WER improves substantially: The best result is attained with the direct method and a 95% artifact threshold, the WER is now only 31.2%: a relative improvement of 13.8%. With backprojection, there is still some improvement, with an optimal WER of 34.2% at an artifact threshold of 80%. However we observe that the direct method works better than backprojection, and that the results between the direct method and backprojection are not fully consistent.

Figure 7.5 summarizes the results of the artifact removal algorithm for the other three setups, again using the respective optimal settings taken from table 7.1 (in particular, for the A-2 setup, no PCA preprocessing is used). We see that the encouraging results from the B-1 setup do *not* carry over to other configurations: In particular, for the 16-channel array, ICA application causes the WER to increase, and removing ICA channels does not improve the results either. This is not the case for setup B, yet for the 160-channel system, we do not observe improvement by application of the artifact removal algorithm either.

Finally, we report on the performance of the artifact removal algorithm on the *evaluation* part of the EMG-ARRAY corpus. Since our experiments so far do not show a consistent improvement when applying the algorithm, we refrain from stating a statistical hypothesis at this point.

We run two experiments, as before: In the first step, we only consider the *audible* EMG. In a second step, we train and evaluate multi-mode systems. In all cases, we use the optimal PCA settings from table 7.1.

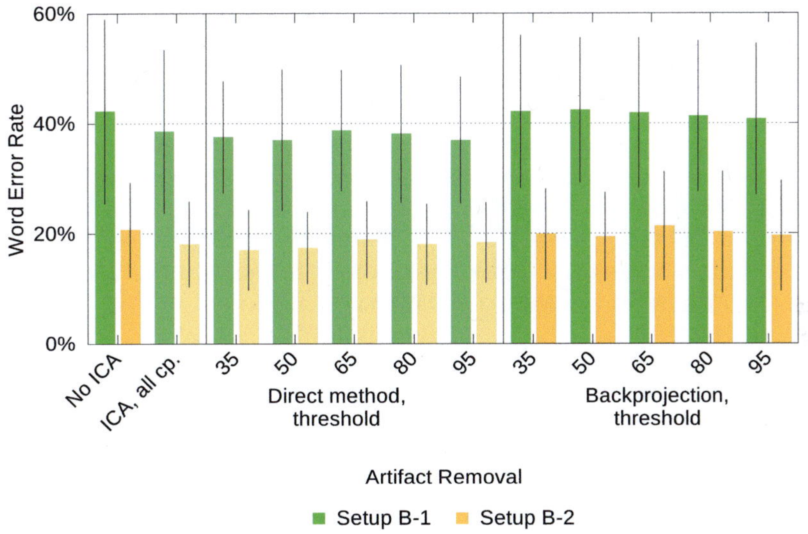

Figure 7.6 – Average Word Error Rates of the ICA-based artifact removal algorithm with different artifact thresholds on the audible part of the EMG-ARRAY *evaluation* corpus. We used optimal PCA settings. Bars indicate standard deviation.

Figure 7.6 displays the average Word Error Rates with ICA application and artifact removal on the audible part of the EMG-ARRAY evaluation corpus. We see that contrary to the results on the development corpus, the artifact removal algorithm yields improvements on both the B-1 and B-2 setup when applied according to the direct method. Backprojection yields higher WERs. The result is not consistent across the setups: For the B-1 setup, an artifact threshold of 95% is optimal, for the B-2 setup, a 35% threshold is substantially better.

Setup	B-1		B-2	
Tested on	Aud. EMG	Sil. EMG	Aud. EMG	Sil. EMG
No Spectral Mapping				
WER without ICA	41.0%	70.6%	24.6%	63.7%
WER with ICA (all comp.)	33.6%	72.0%	21.2%	58.6%
WER with ICA and artifact removal (95% / 35% thr.)	37.3%	68.0%	20.8%	56.0%
With Spectral Mapping				
WER without ICA	40.8%	67.9%	26.4%	56.2%
WER with ICA (all comp.)	36.8%	68.6%	22.3%	55.5%
WER with ICA and artifact removal (95% / 35% thr.)	35.8%	66.1%	23.1%	53.8%

Table 7.4 – Word Error Rates for the ICA-based artifact removal algorithm on multi-mode systems. All systems used optimal settings according to table 7.1, the artifact threshold was set to 95% for the B-1 setup and 35% for the B-2 setup.

Finally, table 7.4 summarizes the performance of the artifact removal algorithm on the *multi-mode* systems trained based on the evaluation corpus. We compare three experiments, namely, no ICA application, ICA application without channel removal ("all components"), and ICA plus artifact removal according to the optimal settings taken from figure 7.6, i.e. direct method with a 95% resp. 35% threshold. Also, Spectral Mapping is additionally applied.

We see that in all cases, the WER with artifact removal is substantially lower than without any ICA application. However, in some cases simple ICA application performs even better. So we conclude that while application of ICA, with or without detection and removal of noise channels, is frequently helpful for obtaining a better signal representation, it is not yet clear what exactly makes this representation good, and how to obtain consistent results.

Future work will further investigate this issue, particularly in light of improved signal decomposition methods. It will also be necessary to reconsider the interplay of the various signal and feature processing steps which are part of our setup, i.e. ICA, PCA, and LDA: In [WHH$^+$13, WJH$^+$ar], we reported substantially better performance for the ICA-based artifact removal algorithm; the major difference between those experiments and the ones reported in this thesis is the lower number of retained dimensions after LDA (12 versus 32). It is certainly possible that a more restrictive LDA dimensionality reduction also helps to remove artifacts at feature level, which might explain why in some cases, particularly for the 16-channel setup A, the ICA-based artifact removal step as applied in this thesis did not improve the average WER of our systems towards the baseline.

7.5 Summary

This chapter introduced our new EMG recording system based on electrode arrays. Our first step was the establishment of a baseline recognition setup, which uses two EMG arrays with a total of 35 channels recorded in bipolar derivation. Here we showed that PCA application is required as an additional preprocessing step in order to allow good LDA estimation.

The first concrete application of the array-based recording setup is an artifact removal algorithm based on Independent Component Analysis (ICA). In the majority of the experiments we ran, we obtain substantially improved Word Error Rates compared to the baseline system without ICA application. Yet, we observed that these improvements are not consistent, which hints to the necessity of further research, particularly with respect to signal transformations: First, the interplay of ICA, PCA, and LDA is to be studied, second, improved source separation and localization methods might bring further accuracy gains.

Even though the results of applying our ICA-based artifact removal algorithm are somewhat inconsistent, we consider the approach a success nonetheless: It proves that information can be extracted from EMG array recordings which is not available in the classical single-channel setup. It is clear from the definition of ICA that there is no point in applying it to the EMG signals from the single-channel setup, since in that case, the captured sources are too diverse, and the number of EMG channels too low, to obtain a sensible signal source decomposition. (We did some side experiments in this regard, which verified this assumption.) So we conclude that the EMG array recordings contain information which the classical EMG-PIT and EMG-UKA corpora do not contain, and which can be used to improve EMG-based speech recognition. With the experiments in this chapter, we have laid a foundation for such experiments, and we leave it to future research to build on these results.

Chapter 8

Applying EMG-based Speech Recognition

This chapter describes necessary steps towards deploying the EMG-based speech recognizer in a practical scenario. We consider ***session independency*** *to be a major step towards real-world usability of the system: a session-independent recognizer may be trained by a user at his or her convenience, and can then be applied without further enrollment whenever the need arises to communicate silently. We show that session-independent systems exhibit quite satisfactory performance, which can be further improved by online* ***adaptation*** *of the system. Speaker independency is also considered, however such systems are not yet ready for practical usage.*

As a proof of the real-world usability of EMG-based speech recognition, and as an application of the results obtained in this thesis, an online demonstration system was created, using many of the algorithms and techniques devised in this thesis.

Whenever a new technology emerges, the question of practical applicability arises both from the general public and from the scientific community. We believe that Silent Speech interfaces have the potential to revolutionize assistive technologies for speech-disabled patients, as well as to greatly reduce the inherent problems of conventional speech communication in public places, i.e. compromised privacy, disturbance of the environment, and susceptibility to environmental noise. Among Silent Speech processing technologies, the EMG approach is considered to have great potential [DSH$^+$10].

The goal of this thesis is not only to develop algorithms and methods which improve the "offline" recognition of pre-recorded silent speech, but also to work towards application of the technology in real-life scenarios. This influenced the research conducted in this thesis, as follows: First, issues which might impede practical usage of EMG-based speech recognition were to be identified and resolved, and second, a quick and powerful demonstration system was to be developed.

Which are the issues when applying our system in practice? From a user's perspective, we identified the following major points:

- Quick setup and ease of use: The attachment of electrodes should be possible very quickly, ideally taking just as long as it normally takes to answer a (mobile) phone call. The risk of mistakes (wrong attachment, bad electrode-skin contact, etc.) should be low.
- Low intrusiveness: Using the system should not induce discomfort to the user.
- Fast enrollment: As most machine learning technologies, EMG-based speech recognition requires a training phase before being usable. It is desired to minimize the required amount of user-specific training, especially immediately before use.
- Robustness: The system should be as robust as possible, and it should degrade gracefully in the presence of errors. Robustness includes dealing with varying environmental conditions and situations, as well as different speaking or articulation styles.
- Flexibility: As few constraints as possible should be imposed on the user.

Furthermore, questions of pricing and availability play a role. While EMG-based continuous speech recognizers are not yet commercially available, their market potential has been judged positively e.g. by [DSH+10]. We do not elaborate on this topic here.

This thesis addresses the above issues in the following ways.

- A system which is quickly and easily set up is provided by the array-based recording apparatus presented in chapter 7. The experience of our recorded subjects, as well as of the student assistants who supervised these recordings, suggest a clear improvement over the old, single-electrode setup: Instead of identifying positions for around 10 single electrodes, it is now only necessary to affix two arrays. Additionally, it becomes much easier to correct misplacements at the algorithmic level, research on this topic is just underway [WSJS14]. Dry EMG electrode arrays, which are already commercially available e.g. by *OT Biolettronica*, are expected to be used in the future and will eliminate contact problems related to gelled electrodes (drying-out, bad application of the gel, etc.).

- EMG-based Silent Speech capturing is judged quite convenient, for example by [DSH$^+$10]; in particular, the system is portable and very lightweight. Note that portable amplifiers which allow to capture a large number of channels and can work with the EMG arrays are available, even though they have not been used for this thesis.
  Nonetheless it is clear that further improvement in usability and user comfort is desired. Our users sometimes found it disconcerting that conductive gel needs to be applied to the electrodes. The array-based recording system offers a partial remedy: here the electrode gel is replaced by an *electrolyte cream*, which feels similar to standard skin cream and is therefore much more agreeable than standard medical-purpose gel. As mentioned above, future efforts will include using *dry* electrodes, which may be held onto the face without requiring gel.

- Fast enrollment of the system may have several meanings. In the optimal case, a speaker could apply the system out-of-the-pocket, without any need for training: This would mean creating *speaker-independent* models. We found it more applicable to train *session-independent* systems, where a speaker pre-trains the system at an arbitrary time, and the system can then be applied without any need for recording further training samples. Session-independency is an issue because applying the system means attaching the electrodes; so far we do not expect a user to wear the EMG electrodes continuously. Differences in electrode positioning, skin properties, and environmental conditions may degrade session-independent systems. Fast enrollment by session independency and session adaptation is the major technical achievement presented in this chapter, leading towards our online demonstration system.

- Robustness is a goal in all experiments conducted for this thesis. A direct measure of robustness is the Word Error Rate, yet we note in passing that recognition errors may have different impact on the understanding of the recognized speech: A wrongly recognized function word, like an article, hardly matters, whereas errors on content-bearing words are much more serious. We do not pursue this topic here, our definition of "robustness" remains as simple as possible: We intend to obtain low Word Error Rates, even under varying conditions.
  So far we have tackled the following aspects. BDPF modeling, presented in chapter 5, yielded a general improvement of recognition rates. Robustness

in *multi-mode* scenarios where the audible, whispered, and silent speaking mode are mixed has been dealt with in chapter 6, where the Spectral Mapping algorithm was introduced. Artifact suppression is one application of the EMG array technology presented in chapter 7. Below, we deal with robustness across *sessions* and *speakers*: When the electrodes are removed or reattached, or when training and test data stem from different speakers, recognition results degrade. Session *independency* and *adaptation* are shown to successfully address this problem. Speaker independency cannot yet be achieved without a substantial loss of accuracy.
Still, speech recognition is not expected to yield completely error-free results in conversational, unplanned speech. One possible remedy for this issue is to apply a direct synthesis of speech signals from EMG, bypassing vocabulary and language modeling issues. We conducted several initial experiments, outside the scope of this thesis [TWS09, NJWS11, JWNS12] (co-work with Matthias Janke), showing that this approach is feasible. We observed that errors in the synthesis cause a degradation of the output speech, but that the content and intended meaning often remain understandable.

- So far, the system's flexibility is somewhat limited due to the fixed 108-word vocabulary which has been used in all previous experiments. We will see that this limit can be raised when a larger amount of training data is used, and indeed, beyond fast enrollment, the session-independent systems presented in this chapter allow using much more training data than is available for the session-dependent systems. This enables us to use an enlarged vocabulary of 2102 words for the experiments presented below.

This chapter is structured as follows: In the first section 8.1 we report on our experiments on session-independent modeling, which is understood as combining different sessions of *one and the same* speaker. Results on speaker-independent systems are also reported, although they are less promising than the session-independent approach.

We then consider session *adaptation*, where a session-independent *background* system is adapted towards a new *target* session with a small amount of *adaptation* data: In section 8.2 we show that adaptation further improves the recognition accuracy, even when the content of the adaptation data is unknown (*unsupervised adaptation*). Thus the issue of fast enrollment is addressed.

Finally, in section 8.3 we present our online demonstration system, which uses session adaptation as a key component.

8.1 Recognition Across Multiple Sessions and Speakers

8.1.1 Session-independent Systems

Session-independent (SI) systems are characterized by using a large number of recording sessions from one and the same speaker for training and testing, so that the sets of training and test sessions are disjoint. The *multi-session* part of the EMG-UKA corpus, consisting of audible EMG data from 32 sessions of speaker 2 and 16 sessions of speaker 8, provides the means to conduct such experiments. Experiments on the array-based system are not performed since there are not enough sessions per speaker available.

EMG-based speech recognition across multiple sessions was first reported on in the extensive works of L. Maier-Hein [MHMSW05, MH05a], but only for a whole-word recognition task. We presented initial results on session-independent (and session-adaptive) training of BDPF models in [WS11b], using a subset of the corpus used in this chapter.

We use SI systems based on 7 or 15 training sessions. Seven-session systems are created in the following way:

- The 32 sessions of speaker 2 are divided into four blocks of eight sessions. The 16 sessions of speaker 8 are divided into two blocks of eight sessions.
- We train and test eight systems on each block with a leave-one-out pattern, i.e. each system is trained on seven of the sessions and tested on the remaining session, which we designate the *target* session. Altogether we obtain 48 systems, each with a different target session out of the 48 sessions in the multi-mode EMG-UKA corpus. Each such system is trained on the $7 \cdot 40 = 280$ training utterances of 7 sessions.

SI systems based on 15 training sessions are created similarly, using two blocks of 16 sessions for speaker 2 and one block of 16 sessions for speaker 8. For each block we trained 16 systems with a leave-one-out pattern, the resulting 48 systems each receive $15 \cdot 40 = 600$ training utterances.

The sessions are sorted in chronological order of recording, i.e. the sessions of the second block were recorded *after* all sessions of the first block, and so on. All experiments are based on the optimal BDPF system from chapter 5, since only audible EMG data is used, the Spectral Mapping algorithm described in chapter 6 is not applicable. Also note that the LDA transformation is computed on the training data set of each system, in particular, there is only one LDA transformation for each trained system. As we saw in chapter 7, the LDA estimation is susceptible to the amount of data used for its estimation. However, we do not pursue this issue here, since the data dimensionality is small, and the amount of training data is larger than in our baseline session-dependent system, so that singularity issues are not expected. We do, however, reconsider the number of retained features after LDA application. Here we may expect that the optimal number of features rises when more training data is available.

It is also clear that a larger amount of training data yields better recognition results. Below, we compare the 7-session and 15-session SI systems and show that this is indeed the case. Since SI training gives us the chance to work with vastly more data than in the session-dependent *(SD)* setup, we can perform recognition experiments on an extended vocabulary consisting of 2102 words: This is the entire set of words from the EMG-UKA corpus, denoted the *Full* vocabulary. Enlarging the recognition vocabulary is very important with respect to the usability of the system, since a vocabulary of 108 words only allows rather elementary communication, whereas the enlarged vocabulary should be sufficient for a basic conversation. We refer to the original 108-word vocabulary, which is still used for comparison, as *Base* vocabulary. For the experiments on unsupervised adaptation, we additionally need a smaller, session-dependent vocabulary (the *Spec* vocabulary), see section 8.2.3.

We frequently compare the SI systems to the 48 session-dependent baseline systems available from the multi-session part of the EMG-UKA corpus. It should be noted that this comparison is valid since the test sets of these systems are identical (all testing is done on the BASE data of the multi-mode part of the EMG-UKA corpus).

The first experiment deals with finding optimal parameters for the SI systems. Figure 8.1 presents the average Word Error Rates of the four setups, differing in the decoding vocabulary and in the amount of training data (7 or 15 sessions). On the horizontal axis of each plot, the number of retained components after the LDA step is charted.

We first observe that for both the SI and SD case, increasing the amount of words in the decoding vocabulary yields a substantial loss of accuracy. In terms of LDA application, by comparing figures 4.5 and 8.1 it is immediately observed that the results differ from the SD baseline system, where the optimal number of retained components was 12: This number is suboptimal for the SI systems, the optimum is reached at around 16 – 24 LDA components. Since two of the systems (the best one, with 15 training sessions and a 108-word decoding vocabulary, and the worst one, with 7 training sessions and 2102-word decoding vocabulary) attain optimal performance at 24 LDA components, we choose this number for all further experiments on session-independent and session-adaptive recognition.

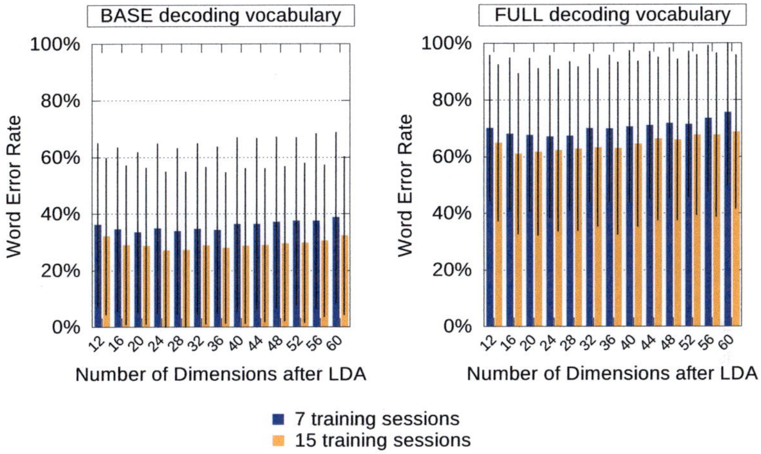

Figure 8.1 – Average Word Error Rates for the session-independent system, versus different numbers of retained features after LDA, decoding with the *Base* vocabulary (left) and the *Full* vocabulary (right). Bars indicate standard deviation.

Note that we still use 12 LDA components for the session-dependent systems which are used for comparison. This approach is considered valid since for the comparison between two setups with vastly different training data conditions, an "one-size-fits-all" philosophy is clearly wrong and would lead to an unfair comparison between the different systems, no matter whether the smaller or greater dimensionality might be chosen. Instead, we run each experiment with its optimal settings.

With our parameters fixed, we now turn to comparing the different recognition setups. Figure 8.2 compares the WERs of the SD system and the two SI systems *by block*, i.e. averages have been taken over the eight-session blocks described above. The average WERs are also given, they are additionally summarized in table 8.1.

It can be seen that in the majority of cases, SI systems trained on 15 sessions yield almost as good recognition as the SD systems, *without* using any training data of the target session at all. For some blocks, the 15-session SI systems even outperform the SD systems, however on blocks 3 and 4 of speaker 2, the SI systems do not perform well. This hints to unusually high variations in recording conditions between these sessions, possibly because their recording spread over several months—during this time, tiny variations in electrode positioning might

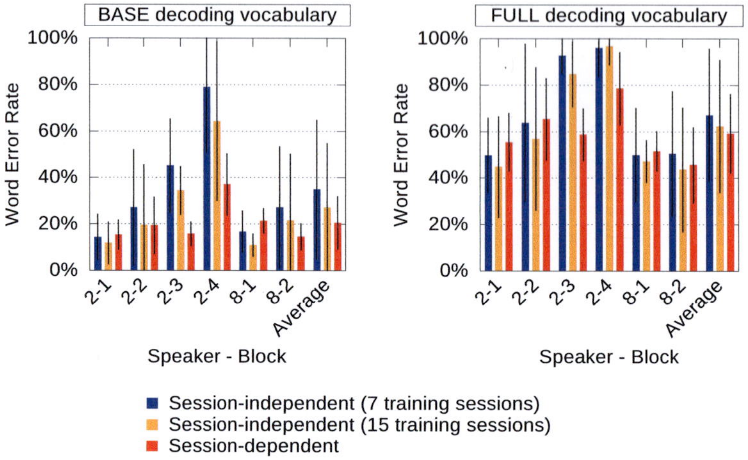

Figure 8.2 – Average Word Error Rates for the session-independent systems, broken down by blocks. Bars indicate standard deviation.

have remained undetected. It is also clear that the systems improve when the number of training sessions is increased. We also made this (expected) observation for session-dependent systems [WS11b].

From these results, we can draw the conclusion that session-independent recognition works well, as long as it is assured that recording conditions match. A mismatch between recording conditions is clearly present in blocks 3 and 4 of speaker 2: This went undetected during our data corpus collection, since we did not run the recognizer during our offline recordings. However, in a practical setting the user would immediately notice such a mismatch, so that for example, the array positioning could be corrected.

The impact of this result on practical applications is high: Now a speaker may pre-train his or her system at any point prior to usage, and then apply it without further enrollment. There remains the open question whether it is necessary to record *multiple* recording sessions in order to make the system robust with respect to a new session (by definition, a setup using data from one single session for training and another session for testing is also session-independent). Presumably, using more training sessions allows the models to represent a larger variation in recording conditions, which should yield more stable behavior towards session variations in the test data.

Setup	Average WER and standard deviation	
	Base decoding vocabulary	*Full* decoding vocabulary
SI (7 sessions)	34.9% ± 29.9%	67.1% ± 28.5%
SI (15 sessions)	27.0% ± 27.8%	62.3% ± 28.5%
SD	20.5% ± 11.3%	59.2% ± 17.0%

Table 8.1 – Word Error Rates and standard deviations for different setups and both decoding vocabularies

The above experiments do not answer this question, since between the 7-session and 15-session SI systems, we increased the amount of training data and the number of training sessions simultaneously. Therefore as a last experiment in SI recognition, we investigate to what extent the number of training sessions influences the recognition results *when the amount of training data is kept fixed.*

We employ the following setups:

- Systems are trained on 120 utterances, using 3 to 7 sessions from one 8-session block for training, and one of the remaining sessions for testing.
- Systems are trained on 180 utterances, using 6 to 15 sessions from one 16-session block for training, and one of the remaining sessions for testing.

This means that only a subset of the SPEC training data of each session is taken; this subset is randomly selected. When less than 7 resp. 15 sessions are used for training, we follow a fixed pattern to determine which sessions are used. Altogether we obtain 48 systems for each setup, each tested on one of the 48 sessions of our corpus as usual. This makes the results comparable to our prior setup.

Figure 8.3 depicts the WERs with the setups described above, where we performed decoding on the 108-word *Base* vocabulary since the number of training utterances is too small to allow the full 2102-word vocabulary. We see that in general, training on more sessions improves the resulting WER, with one exception (with 180 training sentences, 15 sessions perform slightly worse than 12 sessions).

On the 120-sentence setup, the session-wise difference between the WERs on the 3-session and the 7-session setup is 6.2% (absolute) with a confidence interval ranging from -0.2% to 12.6%, so statistical significance of the resulting improvement is *not* asserted. Similarly, on the 180-sentence setup, the WER difference between the 6-session training and the 15-session training is 4.6% (absolute) with a confidence interval ranging from -1.6% to 10.8%.

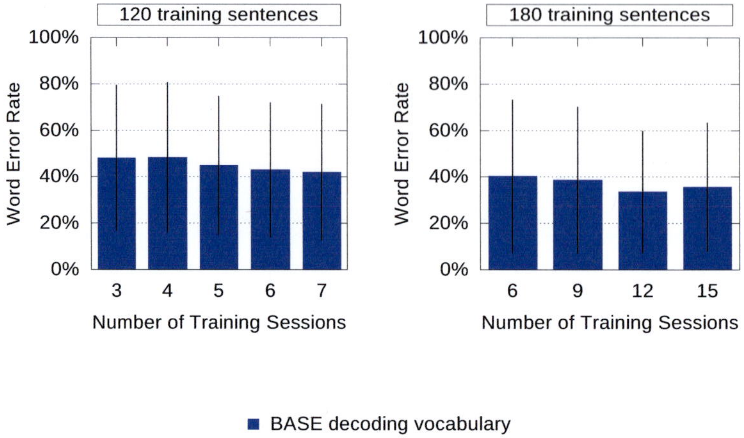

Figure 8.3 – Average Word Error Rates for session-independent systems with a *fixed* amount of training data which is taken from a *varying* number of sessions. Bars indicate standard deviation.

Summarizing our experiments on session indepencency, it is clear that the method works and is feasible. We saw that the SI systems with 15 training sessions almost reach the accuracy of session-dependent systems. 15 training sessions amount to 600 utterances, or around 45 minutes of training data (see table 3.3), which is far more than the training data from the one target session. It appears that the discrepancy between sessions is a major detriment for the recognizer, which requires substantial amounts of data to be compensated for. On the other hand, the ability to deal with unseen sessions is a major benefit, besides improving practical applicability of the system it allows to accrue far more data than could ever be collected in one session. Under suitable circumstances, the required amount of data for session-independent recognition should be available in practice. We will return to this topic below in section 8.2, where we show that session *adaptation* may combine the advantages of SI and SD systems, even in the "unsupervised" case.

8.1.2 Speaker-independent Systems

With session-independent recognition being established, we consider *speaker independency* the next goal. Speaker independency means that a system is tested

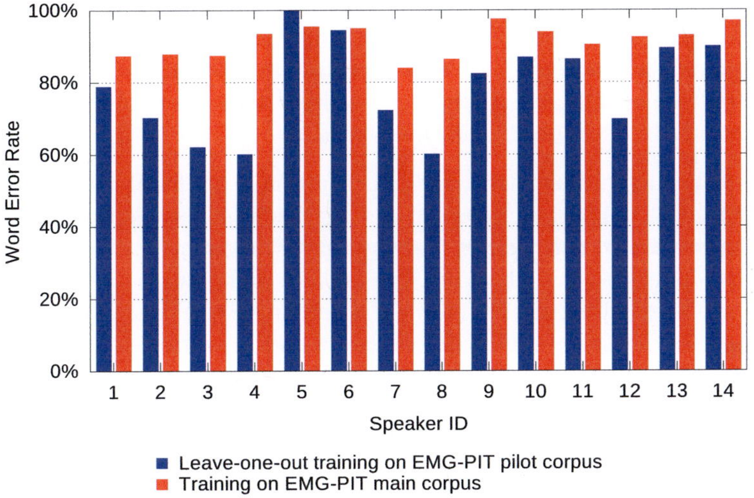

Figure 8.4 – Average Word Error Rates for speaker-independent systems, trained on the EMG-PIT pilot corpus using a leave-one-out setup (training was performed on the 13 speakers who were *not* tested) and on the EMG-PIT main corpus. The 14 test speakers are from the EMG-PIT pilot corpus. All results are on the 108-word *Base* vocabulary.

on data from a speaker who was not part of the training data set: A system working in this way would allow a user to apply an EMG-based silent speech recognizer without any prior training at all.

The EMG-PIT corpus was recorded with the specific purpose of allowing to train systems on data from a large number of speakers. So we base an initial experiment, first reported in [WS09, WS10], on the pilot part of the EMG-PIT corpus, using a leave-one-out method as follows: 14 speaker-independent systems are trained, each using the training data from 13 speakers and the testing data from the remaining speaker, in both cases combining the two sessions from each speaker. As for the experiments on session-independency, we only use audible EMG. We also performed an experiment using *all* the data from the EMG-PIT main corpus for training a speaker-independent system: This amounts to 62 sessions, i.e. more than 4.3 hours of training data. Testing was again performed on the test sets of the pilot speakers. We use the 108-word *Base* vocabulary.

The results of both experiments are charted in figure 8.4. We observe that speaker-independent systems exhibit a drastically higher WER than session-independent systems: No speaker attains less the 60% WER in any experiment.

The average WER is 78.9% for the leave-one-out systems trained on the EMG-PIT pilot corpus, and 91.5% for the system trained on the EMG-PIT main corpus: So using more data for recognizer training causes deteriorating results. We also observe that the results are not consistent: Neither does more training data help, nor can we distinguish "good" and "bad" speakers.

We conclude that speaker-independent recognition is not feasible at this point: The extracted **TD**n features appear to be very much speaker-dependent. However, new insights are to be gained from investigations on the EMG array system: In the near future, we expect clearer insights into different sources of EMG activity, and we expect to have the means of extracting signals from these sources. It may be possible to map such activity sources between different speakers, thus compensating for speaker discrepancies by versatile feature extraction.

8.2 Fast Enrollment by Model Adaptation

In the previous section we showed that session-independent (SI[1]) systems are feasible. However, the SI systems do not reach the full potential of session-dependent (SD) systems: When a system trained on 7 sessions is applied to the test data of an unseen target session, this results in a higher WER than the corresponding session-dependent system, even though the SI system receives seven times more training data than the SD system. With 15 training sessions, the SI systems do improve, but even here we can legitimately assume that SD systems with the same amount of training data would work far better (in [WS11b] we reported on some experiments with different training data sizes for SD and SI systems, clearly showing that both systems improve when more training data is added). Still, we intend session-independent systems to perform as good as possible, since this is a major feature in practical scenarios.

The adaptation algorithms which are described and investigated in this chapter aim at combining the advantageous properties of large "background" systems and small specific systems, where the designations *large* and *small* refer to the available amount of training data. The standard application of adaptation in acoustic speech recognition, from where we take our algorithm, is transforming a large speaker-independent system towards a specific speaker. Here it is clear that the speaker-independent "background" system is much larger than any speaker-specific system. For example, the current version of the well-known *GlobalPhone*

[1]Note that as defined above, the abbreviation *SI* always means "session-independent", not "speaker-independent".

corpus consists of more than 400 hours of transcribed speech data [SVS13], far more than one speaker could ever produce in a supervised setting.

Adaptation has many applications and comes in many flavors. In chapter 6, we presented the *Spectral Mapping* algorithm as a signal-based method adapting silent EMG towards audible EMG, using prior knowledge about the EMG signal properties. In this chapter, we only consider *model* adaptation using the *Maximum Likelihood Linear Regression* (MLLR) algorithm [GW96]: Trained models are adapted to better fit the target data. This kind of adaptation is a form of training, and indeed, MLLR even shares its target function with standard Maximum Likelihood Baum-Welch training, as described below. Further applications of adaptation in speech recognition include gearing a system towards dealing with specific background noise, dialects or accents, etc.; adaptation is also applied increasingly often in other domains, including e-mail spam filtering [BS07] and visual object recognition [SKFD10].

MLLR requires existing pre-trained *background* models, as well as *adaptation* data to reestimate the GMM parameters. In this thesis, adaptation is always performed between sessions, i.e. training, adaptation and test data stem from different sessions, but from the same speaker. Training is performed on the combined SPEC data from several sessions, yielding any of the session-independent systems described in section 8.1.1. Adaptation data comes from the *target* session: the SPEC data of the target session is used for adaptation, and the BASE data is used for evaluating the recognizer, as usual. This makes our systems comparable to session-dependent systems, which are trained on this adaptation data. Adaptation between speakers is not considered due to the low baseline performance of the speaker-independent systems.

Ideally, an adapted system performs better than both the background SI system and the SD system trained on just the adaptation data. Below it is proved that session adaptation indeed improves the recognition accuracy beyond the limits of both session-independent and session-dependent systems. These limits depend, of course, on the available amount of training data, as becomes clear from the results of section 8.1.1: Session-adaptive systems only make sense if the amount of data on which the SI background system is trained is substantially larger than the amount of SD data, otherwise the SD systems perform better.

In the remainder of this section, the theoretical background of the MLLR adaptation method is explained, and the results of applying MLLR are presented.

8.2.1 Review of the MLLR Method

In this section we briefly review the MLLR as it is implemented in our system, mostly based on the classical overview article [GW96] by Gales and Woodland. We compare the concept of adaptation to the standard maximum likelihood training described in section 2.3.5, illustrate the prerequisites and benefits of adaptation, and finally describe the MLLR algorithm.

Gales and Woodland describe the purpose of adaptation as follows ([GW96, Abstract]): "One of the key issues for adaptation algorithms is to modify a large number of parameters with only a small amount of adaptation data." This emphasizes the key concept of adaptation: Pre-existing background models are modified based on some small amount of new adaptation data, and the background system should be *larger* than the system one could create solely from the adaptation data. Indeed, the MLLR algorithm yields no theoretical benefit over EM training if the amount of adaptation data is large, compared to the training data used for the background system. Only if the amount of adaptation data is small, MLLR can play out its strength.

We also see that MLLR requires that background models exist: This is a major difference to the standard training procedure described in section 2.3.5, which creates Gaussian models from scratch.

MLLR as employed here is a *model* adaptation method, which means that the (myoelectric) model is transformed to better match the adaptation data[2]. Thus the Gaussian parameters (means, covariances, and possibly component weights) are updated: MLLR adaptation is a form of *training*, just like standard Baum-Welch training.

For now we make the prerequisite that transcriptions of the adaptation data are available, i.e. their textual content is known. We can additional assume that assignments of feature vectors to HMM states, and to the underlying Gaussian components, have been computed e.g. by the Viterbi algorithm or the Forward-backward algorithm. This means that one could perform one step of EM training at this stage, incurring a recomputation of all Gaussian parameters.

MLLR shares its optimization target function with the EM training described in section 2.3.5, namely, the likelihood of the adaptation data, given by equation 2.4, is to be maximized. However in constrast to Baum-Welch EM training, this is not done by completely replacing the Gaussian parameters: instead a *transformation* of the parameters is estimated, as follows.

[2] A feature-space MLLR [Gal97] also exists and shares some properties with model-space MLLR.

The new mean for a Gaussian component distribution is computed by ([GW96, Chapters 2, 3][3])

$$\hat{\mu} = A\mu + b, \tag{8.1}$$

where the transformation is given by the full matrix A and the bias vector b. μ is the old mean, which is thus linearly transformed. Similarly, the new covariance is computed by the equation ([GW96, Chapter 4])

$$\hat{\Sigma} = B^T H B, \tag{8.2}$$

where H is the estimated transformation, and B is the inverse of the Cholesky factor of the original inverse covariance matrix, i.e. $\Sigma^{-1} = CC^T$ with a lower triangular matrix C having positive diagonal entries, and $B = C^{-1}$. H depends on the newly computed mean $\hat{\mu}$, so that in practice, the update of mean and covariance matrix is done in two steps.

The transformations A, b, and H are computed based on the collected statistics of the adaptation data. For details about their estimation we refer to the original article [GW96]; here we are interested in understanding the properties of the MLLR. As the equations show, the original values of μ and Σ enter the computation of the respective new values (in contrast to standard Baum-Welch training, see equation 2.5). Yet it is clear from equation 8.1 that *any* vector $\hat{\mu}$ can be the result of the linear shift $\hat{\mu} = A\mu + b$, and since A and b are estimated so that the likelihood of the adaptation data is maximized, it follows that naïve application of equation 8.1 yields the same estimate for $\hat{\mu}$ as the Baum-Welch rule given by equation 2.5 does. A similar reasoning holds for the covariance update given by equation 8.2.

Given this observation, why is it sensible to use MLLR at all? When MLLR is applied, the underlying background system is trained with far more data than one may use for the adaptation step. This typically means that the background system has substantially more Gaussians than might properly be trained with the adaptation data, and here the second component of the MLLR concept comes into play: The set of Gaussian component distributions is partitioned into a relatively small number of (disjoint) subsets, and all Gaussians which are members of one such subset are *jointly* transformed, pooling their assigned adaptation data. This allows the reestimation of a large number of Gaussian parameters with a small amount of adaptation data and is the principal reason why MLLR is applicable to adaptation tasks.

In our implementation, the grouping of Gaussians is performed using a binary regression class tree, similar to the principle outlined in [Gal96] (but with a simpler

[3]Gales and Woodland use a slightly different notation, where A and b are combined into one matrix $W = (A|b)$.

splitting criterion). Using a tree structure for determining clusters of Gaussians to be adapted is advantageous because it flexibly accomodates different amounts of adaptation data: This concept already played a role for our recognizer in the BDPF clustering procedure described in section 5.2.2.

The regression class tree is created as follows: First a set of *all* Gaussian component distributions is formed, regardless of the unit model they belong to. This set of all Gaussians is assigned to the regression class tree root node. Now the tree nodes are recursively split as follows: For each node, all mean vectors of the Gaussians contained in this node are considered, and the Gaussians are split into two disjoint groups by running the k-means algorithm with $k = 2$ on the mean vectors. The covariances of the Gaussians are ignored. Finally two child nodes of the original node are created, containing the two subsets of Gaussians created by the k-means algorithm. Now the two child nodes are processed recursively, until the splitting process is stopped at a specific tree depth (for example, at depth 2, four leaf nodes are created).

This regression tree does *not* depend on the adaptation data (which at this stage might not even be available), but only on the models of the background system. Therefore, it is unknown during splitting how much adaptation data will be available for any tree node, or any Gaussian.

When the regression class tree has been computed, adaptation transformations A, b, and H as specified in equations 8.1 and 8.2 are computed for each tree node (including non-leaf nodes). For a node transformation to be computed, it is required that the amount of training data exceeds a certain minimum threshold: Otherwise, no transformation is computed, instead an applicable transformation is searched by ascending the tree until a node with sufficient training data is found.

Figure 8.5 shows an example for such a regression tree: The tree depth, predetermined before adaptation data is even collected, is 2, so we have four leaf nodes. All available Gaussians in the system are partitioned into the disjoint subsets G_4, ..., G_7, and $G_2 = G_4 \uplus G_5$, $G_3 = G_6 \uplus G_7$, $G_1 = G_2 \uplus G_3$. Transformations $W_i = \{A_i, b_i, H_i\}$ have been computed. The partition G_5 did not receive enough adaptation data to exceed the threshold, therefore no transformation was computed here: instead the transformation W_2, which is computed on the *joint* training data from partitions G_4 and G_5, is used for all Gaussians in the partition G_5. Note that the subset G_4 is not affected and uses the transformation W_4.

When transformations have been computed, they are applied to the Gaussian models according to equations 8.1 and 8.2. Note that the mixture weights remain unchanged in our implementation. As for Baum-Welch training, next the assignment of feature frames to Gaussian models can be recomputed, yielding a

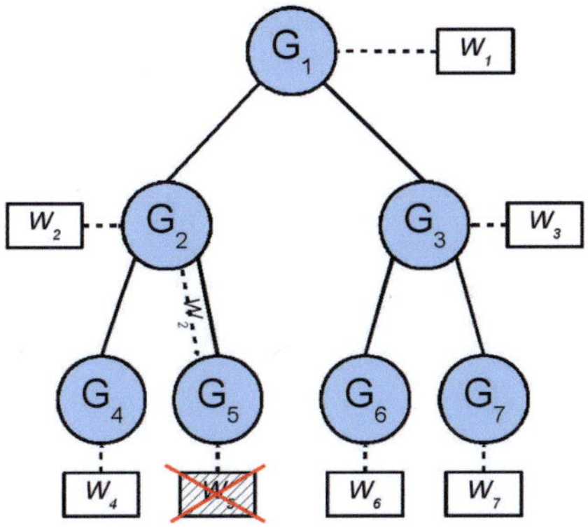

Figure 8.5 – Example MLLR regression tree with depth 2. The node labels G_i indicate a partitioning of the set of all Gaussian component distributions, such that each parent node contains the Gaussians of its child nodes, and no two nodes on the same level share a Gaussian. Each node receives an adaptation transformation W, which is computed on the adaptation data of the assigned Gaussians *if enough adaptation data is available.* In the example, node G_5 does not have enough training data, so the applicable transformation is searched by ascending the tree (in this case, transformation W_2 is found).

typical iterative EM algorithm. When this iteration stops, e.g. after a fixed number of iterations, the recognizer is evaluated as usual on the transformed models.

The algorithm described above is called *supervised* MLLR, since we have adaptation data with accurate phone-level alignments, just as in standard training. The phone-level alignments can be computed from the transcription of the utterance if they are not present, which does not present any problems (this is the *E* step of the EM training of HMMs, performed with the Viterbi algorithm or the forward-backward algorithm, see section 2.3.5). However, if the transcription of an utterance is unavailable, obtaining robust phone-level alignments becomes more challenging.

This situation occurs when ongoing adaptation of the EMG-based speech recognizer is desired even during normal usage. Here EMG data is produced, but the textual content of this data is unknown. Applying adaptation even in this case leads to *unsupervised* MLLR: We assume that we have EMG data for adaptation, but that no transcriptions are available. (Our corpus exclusively contains transcribed data, yet we can of course disregard the transcriptions.)

In order to deal with such a situation, the MLLR algorithm is extended by an additional *decoding* step on the adaptation data, yielding a hypothesized transcription. Of course, some or many of the recognized words might be plainly wrong: Using this hypothesis as a basis for MLLR would possibly deteriorate the model quality instead of enhancing it.

In order to estimate the quality of parts of a hypothesis, *confidence measures* have been developed. These use information from the decoding stage to estimate the probability of recognition errors. We applied a confidence computation method developed by Kemp and Schaaf for acoustic speech recognition, it is the "gamma" method from [KS97].

This confidence computation algorithm is based on *lattices*, which are compact representations of different possible decoding hypotheses in the form of directed graphs: The graph nodes represent words, and edges represent possible successors and predecessors in the set of hypotheses. (Lattices have been developed mainly for performance reasons and memory saving, a list of the n best hypotheses for a given utterance would equally well allow the computation of confidences if n is large enough.)

The words in the lattice are saved together with their (log-)probabilities coming from the myoelectric model and the language model. This means that the total probability of a word at a given timeframe can be computed from the lattice, essentially by applying the forward-backward algorithm at word level. If the probability of a word at a given position in the hypothesis is high, this means that most, or even all, hypotheses from the lattice contain this word at its position. If the word probability is small, the recognizer created many different word hypotheses with similar likelihoods at this timeframe.

These word-level probabilities are used as a confidence measure: When the adaptation transformations A, b, and H are computed, each training data sample is weighted with the local confidence, ranging between 0 (do not use this sample) and 1 (give this sample full weight). No confidence threshold is used. Finally, the estimation of transformations and the update of the Gaussian parameters is performed as in the supervised case.

Good recognition accuracy on the background model is a key prerequisite for using unsupervised adaptation. If the generated hypotheses are not good enough, one will either compute the MLLR based on wrong input transcriptions, thus diminishing the recognition accuracy rather than improving it, or one obtains many low confidences, so that only a small fraction of the training data is used. Also, it is important to optimally tune the recognizer so that best results are obtained.

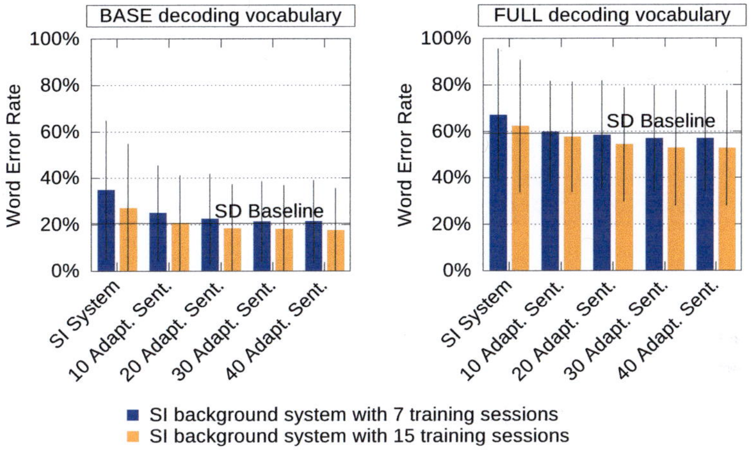

Figure 8.6 – WERs for the session-independent system with different numbers of adaptation sentences for *supervised* adaptation. Bars indicate standard deviation.

8.2.2 Supervised Session Adaptation

In this section we apply the MLLR algorithm for session adaptation in a supervised setting, following our publication [WS11b]. As background systems we use the SI recognizers trained on 7 respectively 15 training data sessions. Adaptation always uses a part of the SPEC sentences of the target session, i.e. the session on which testing is to be performed. We fix the MLLR parameters as follows: The regression tree is computed to a depth of 2, and the minimum amount of adaptation data per node is set to 100 (this is small enough to assure that a transformation can be computed for each node). Four iterations of MLLR training and frame assignment reestimation are performed. We also ran additional experiments with different parameters and found only small variation as long as the parameters remain within a useful range; in particular, increasing the amount of nodes in the adaptation tree does not yield any benefit as long as the amount of adaptation data remains small.

Figure 8.6 shows WERs for the resulting *session-adaptive* systems, for both SI background systems and both decoding vocabularies. The number of adaptation sentences ranges from 10 to 40. We observe that MLLR *always* brings an improvement: Even with only 10 adaptation sentences, the WER decreases drastically, for example, with the 7-session background system and the 108-word

	Decoding vocabulary	
	Base	*Full*
WER improvement: Adaptation versus SI system		
7-session background system	13.6% ± 5.7%	10.2% ± 4.6%
15-session background system	9.6% ± 5.0%	9.6% ± 4.5%
WER improvement: Adaptation versus SD system		
7-session background system	-0.8% ± 3.9%	2.3% ± 5.2%
15-session background system	3.1% ± 3.8%	6.5% ± 5.5%

Table 8.2 – Absolute WER improvements with 95% confidence intervals with supervised session adaptation. The improvement yielded over the session-independent system is significant (the confidence intervals do not contain 0 in all four cases). Significance of the improvement over the *session-dependent* system cannot be asserted.

decoding vocabulary, the WER falls from 34.9% to 25.0%, a relative improvement of 28.4%.

The improvement is greater for larger numbers of adaptation sentences, even though beyond 30 sentences, there emerges a certain saturation effect. With 30 adaptation sentences or beyond, the session-adaptive systems perform better than the SD baseline systems in three out of four cases, which proves the robustness of the session-adaptive systems: We consider this a very important result regarding future practical application of the EMG-based speech recognizer.

Finally, in order to validate the results we computed confidence intervals for the improvements obtained by the MLLR algorithm, using the full 40-sentence adaptation data. Note that for this experiment, a separate evaluation set is unavailable, so that this validation has to be performed on the same 48 sessions on which we optimized our setup.

Table 8.2 shows the *absolute* WER improvements when comparing the MLLR system to the SI and SD systems. It can be seen that the confidence intervals for the improvements of the MLLR system over to the SI system are substantially beyond 0 for all four combinations of decoding vocabulary and background system, so we conclude that the positive effect of MLLR is indeed significant.

When comparing the MLLR system and the session-dependent system, the MLLR system may perform worse than the SD system: this occurs for the 7-session background system and the *Base* decoding vocabulary. In the other cases, we obtain slight improvements, but table 8.2 shows that so far, we cannot conclude that these improvements are sigificant.

	Decoding vocabulary	
	Base	*Full*
WER improvement: *Unsupervised* Adaptation versus SI system		
7-session background system	4.7% ± 2.2%	6.0% ± 3.2%
15-session background system	3.8% ± 1.8%	6.0% ± 2.7%

Table 8.3 – Absolute WER improvements with 95% confidence intervals of unsupervised session adaptation over the session-independent systems. Significance of the improvement can be asserted since all confidence intervals are beyond zero.

8.2.3 Unsupervised Session Adaptation

The final adaptation experiments deal with *unsupervised* session adaptation. We use exactly the same adaptation data as above, however we assume that this data is not transcribed, i.e. its content is unknown. This would by the typical situation when the data has been accrued during practical usage of the system.

As described in section 8.2.1, one can use such utterances for adaptation by performing a decoding step to generate hypotheses and, consequently, phone-level time-alignments. Confidences are used to estimate which parts of a hypothesis are probably correct and should be used for adaptation.

In order to decode the adaptation data, i.e. the SPEC data of the target sessions, we cannot use the *Base* vocabulary since it only contains the words appearing in the BASE test set (see section 4.1.4). Therefore we define a new type of vocabulary for the purpose of decoding adaptation data. We call it the *Spec* vocabulary, it is *session-dependent* and contains all words appearing in the SPEC data of the respective session. The number of words in the *Spec* vocabulary varies between 259 and 311, with an average of 299, so the *Spec* vocabulary is almost three times larger than the 108-word *Base* vocabulary which we used in all experiments presented so far for decoding the BASE set.

Figure 8.7 charts the WERs for unsupervised adaptation, as well as for the original SI systems and supervised adaptation. For both supervised and unsupervised MLLR, the entire SPEC set of the target session is used for adaptation. We see that unsupervised MLLR indeed brings improvement: For 7-session background training, the WER on the BASE evaluation data drops from 34.9% to 30.2% (13.5% relative improvement) when decoded with the *Base* vocabulary, and from 67.1% to 61.1% (8.9% relative improvement) on the *Full* vocabulary. Similar improvements are observed on the 15-session background systems.

Table 8.3 shows the average absolute improvements for each of the four possible setups, with confidence intervals. All improvements are significant, since the

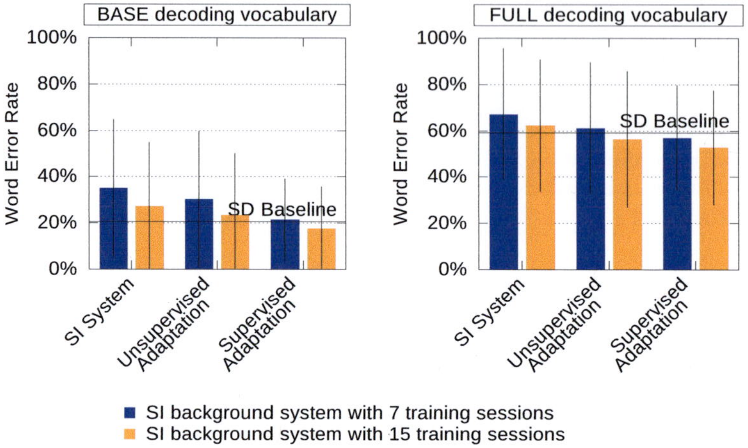

Figure 8.7 – WER comparison for unsupervised and supervised MLLR adaptation with 40 adaptation sentences. In all unsupervised MLLR experiments, the session-dependent *Spec* vocabulary was used for decoding the adaptation data. The BASE evaluation set was decoded with the 108-word *Base* or 2102-word *Full* vocabulary as indicated.

confidence intervals do not contain zero. However, it is clear from figure 8.7 that supervised MLLR is still far better than unsupervised adaptation.

In order to gain understanding of the system, we inspected the hypotheses which are generated during the decoding of the adaptation data. These hypotheses are by no means free of errors: On the adaptation data, the average WER is 44.4% on the 7-session background system and 40.2% on the 15-session background system. Note that these WERs are expected to be higher than on the BASE evaluation set, since the *Spec* vocabulary is larger than the *Base* decoding vocabulary.

Figure 8.8 shows an example of a typical hypothesis of the first session of speaker 2, whose WER on the test data is reduced from 34.30% to 26.30% by unsupervised MLLR. Here the reference is “The federal aviation administration is fiercely defending its operations in testimony before congress”, the hypothesis on the unadapted system is “The federal aviation administration is fiercely defending its operations in testimony *more card is*”, so the last three words are wrongly decoded. Since the reference contains 13 words, and we have two substitutions and one insertion between the reference and the hypothesis, the WER of this particular utterance is thus $\frac{3}{13} \approx 23\%$. We see from figure 8.8 that indeed, the

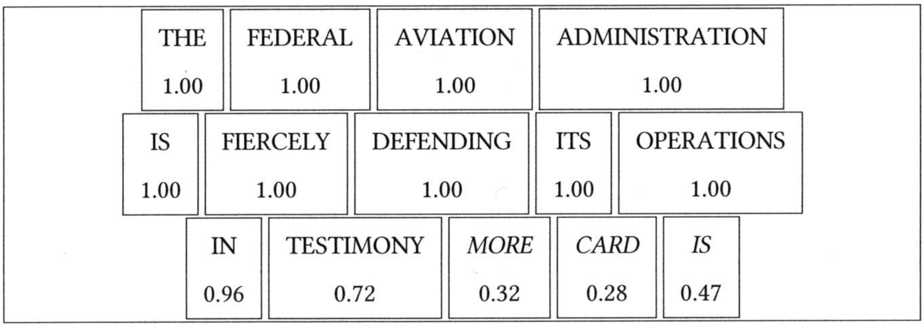

Figure 8.8 – Example hypothesis during unsupervised adaptation, with confidences. The reference was "The federal aviation administration is fiercely defending its operations in testimony before congress", so the last three words were wrongly recognized. They exhibit lower confidence levels than the correctly recognized part of the utterance.

last three words receive far lower confidence probabilities than the first part of the utterance, so the MLLR algorithm will "do the right thing".

It can be said that using confidences incurs a loss of data. This is caused by the way confidences are folded into the accumulation of statistics for MLLR (see section 8.2.1): A sample is weighted (multiplied) with its confidence, so formally, a sample with a confidence smaller than 1.0 is only *partially* used for the computation. This contrasts with the supervised case, where each sample is fully used. On average, in the unsupervised case the 7-session SI background system causes only 8156 frames per PF stream to be accumulated, whereas the supervised system uses the total of 10737 frames (not counting "silence" frames). When the background system is trained on 15 sessions, 8244 frames per stream are used.

From figure 8.2, we observed that there are some sessions which perform very badly ($\approx$ 80% WER) on the SI system. Here unsupervised adaptation usually does not improve the results either, since the background system is too bad to allow creating good hypotheses. However when supervised MLLR is used, or when a session-dependent system is trained, these sessions perform quite well. This is one reason why the average WER improvement of supervised MLLR is well beyond the improvement obtained by unsupervised MLLR: A bad match between background system and adaptation data thus precludes using unsupervised MLLR. A working real-life system could in the future avoid this problem by immediately warning the speaker that the recording setup needs to be fixed.

In the last experiment, we again direct our attention to the question of practical applicability. So far, we used the small *Spec* vocabulary for decoding the adap-

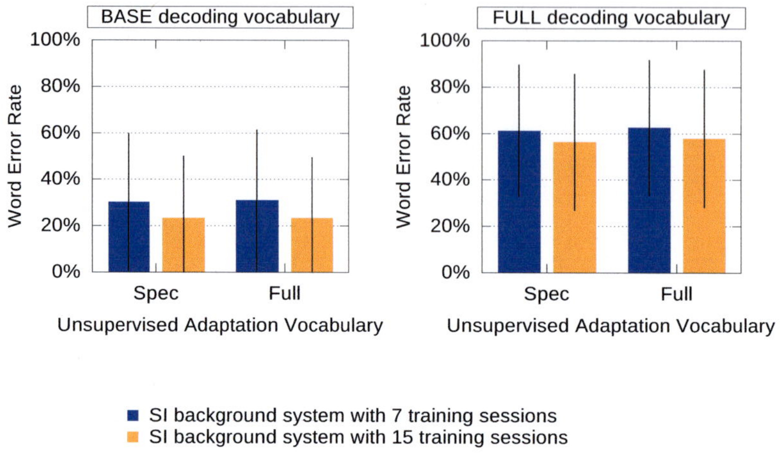

Figure 8.9 – Word Error Rates for unsupervised adaptation using the session-dependent *Spec* vocabulary and the vastly larger *Full* vocabulary. The results only deteriorate very slightly. Bars indicate standard deviation.

tation data: As described above, this means that a speaker would be constrained to using this vocabulary if adaptation data is to be collected. In real-world situations, a larger vocabulary is desired, so we now use the *Full* 2102-word vocabulary not only for system evaluation, but also for decoding the adaptation data. This agrees with practical usage, because the adaptation data will in the future be collected during normal usage of the system: In such a case, the allowable vocabulary should be as large as possible.

Figure 8.9 charts the WER on the BASE evaluation set for different systems using unsupervised MLLR. Somewhat surprisingly, when the full 2102-word vocabulary is used, the resulting WERs only deteriorate very slightly: For example, with the 7-session background system, the WER rises from 30.2% to 31.0% resp. 61.1% to 62.5% when evaluation is performed with the 108-word (*Base*) resp. 2102-word (*Full*) vocabulary.

This is convincing evidence for the robustness of the confidence computation: Accumulation of adaptation statistics works even though the decoding of the adaptation data becomes much harder. The latter reflects in the WER on the adaptation data, which rises from 44.4% to 53.0% on the 7-session background system and from 40.2% to 50.6% on the 15-session background system. Consequently confidences are lower for the *Full* vocabulary decoding than for *Spec* vocabulary decoding, we observe that on average only 7192 resp. 7204 frames are used for adapting the 7 resp. 15 session background system when decoding uses the *Full* vocabulary, compared to 8156 resp. 8244 frames when the adaptation data is decoded with the *Spec* vocabulary. We conclude that even though the WER on the *Full* vocabulary of 2102 words is still relatively high, using this vocabulary does allow the use of the unsupervised adaptation algorithm, which is a key prerequisite when the method is to be used in a real-life setting.

8.2.4 Summary of Adaptation Experiments

In this section, we introduced session-independent (SI) systems and showed that they perform well: With 600 training utterances from 15 sessions, the accuracy of session-independent systems comes close to the one of our session-dependent systems. We then convincingly showed that MLLR-based session adaptation is feasible for EMG-based speech recognition and yields significant improvements over unadapted session-independent systems.

In all experiments, a key issue was the amount of available data: We saw that the performance of session-independent systems, as well as the quality of adaptation, increases when more data is available for training or reestimating models. Standard Baum-Welch training, as well as supervised MLLR adaptation, require transcribed training data: The textual content of this data must be known. Usually, such data is recorded in a controlled setting, i.e. the user reads a series of predetermined text prompts, as described in section 3.2.

Such training data is "expensive": Particularly when speaker-specific systems are desired, each user would have to invest time and care to record his or her own data set. Speaker-independent systems, pre-trained by professional speakers, would offer a remedy here, but we saw that these are not good enough yet.

Here unsupervised adaptation comes into play: This approach is the only training method considered in this thesis which does *not* require that the content of the adaptation data is known. So adaptation data could be collected during normal usage of the EMG-based speech recognizer, allowing to obtain substantially more data than in a controlled setting, without *any* effort of the user.

Unsupervised adaptation clearly does not yet reach the full potential of supervised adaptation, but this *does not matter*: First, significantly more data can be used, and second, the better the underlying system becomes, the better the adaptation works. Thus a recognizer using unsupervised adaptation improves continuously, provided that the original background system is good enough.

It is a very important result that unsupervised adaptation even works with a relatively large underlying vocabulary of more than 2000 words, since this allows useful communication. Clearly, 2000 words is not an upper bound: When even more training data of a speaker has been accumulated (say, several hours), we can legitimately expect far better recognition performance, and far larger allowable vocabularies, than we obtained so far. Also, unsupervised adaptation would continuously update the system when signal properties change during long-term usage (e.g. the skin properties, as well as articulation style, might change over the course of months or even years). Altogether, we conclude that despite some limitations, session-independent and session-adaptive systems provide a powerful means to bridge the gap between research-oriented experiments as presented in chapters 4 – 7, and future practical usage of the system.

8.3 A Real-Time Demonstration System

The final section of this thesis presents an online, real-time demonstration system which has been developed based on the algorithms and methods established in this thesis. We summarize the structure and assembly of the system, give a usage example, and finally summarize insights and experiences gained from the public outreach generated by our demonstrations.

8.3.1 Introduction

The creation of a prototype system was planned right from the beginning of this thesis, and it was tackled as soon as the first major result, the Bundled Phonetic Feature modeling, was achieved. The prototype serves the purpose of proving the validity of our method to the interested public, but also as a means of understanding real-life issues regarding the usage of our system. So far, it is based on the six-channel single-electrode setup—an array-based system is in preparation, however since the EMG-USB2 amplifier, which is currently used for array recordings, is not portable, we only expect to present this system at a later stage, when a mobile recording device will have been integrated.

The prototype is not the first one of its kind: S. Jou, who developed the initial phone-based myoelectric speech recognizer as part of his PhD thesis, developed an initial demonstration for his recognizer, winning the 2006 Interspeech demo award [Jou08]. Our prototype substantially improves this original system, in particular by using the newly developed Bundled Phonetic Feature modeling (see chapter 5), and by allowing continuous recognition in a session-adaptive scenario. These methodological improvements result in a much higher recognition accuracy, which allows us to define a much more complex recognition task than in the prior system.

Our prototype features two demonstration scenarios: The first scenario allows to utter freely formed sentences from the Broadcast News domain, constrained only by the 108-word vocabulary which we use for our standard decoding experiments on the EMG-UKA corpus, described in section 4.1.4. Even though the Broadcast News domain is not a typical domain which we expect to play a role in practical applications, we chose it as the basis of this demonstration system since we have large matching background corpora: So a good fit between training, adaptation, and test sentences is guaranteed.

In order to create a scenario which better matches possibly uses of the system, we created a second setup, based on sentences which might be uttered in a typical silent phone call. Switching between the two scenarios is possible at any time, implying that both demo scenarios share the same training. Thus we have a mismatch between the training/adaptation data and the test data in this case: This is alleviated by using a *context-free grammar* to structure the possible set of utterances; an example conversation mimicking a silent phone call might proceed as follows:

> *Caller:* Good afternoon. Do you have a minute for talking?
> *Silent Speaker:* Good afternoon. Yes, I am sitting in a meeting.
> *Caller:* Uh, but you are able to speak?
> *Silent Speaker:* Yes, since I am using my new Silent Speech recognizer. I can talk to you by simply mouthing words.
> *Caller:* Oh, OK. When should we meet in person?
> *Silent Speaker:* A good time would be seven o'clock. Let us have dinner at a restaurant.
> *Caller:* This would be fine with me.
> *Silent Speaker:* Great, see you there.

Here the silent speaker would be able to modify the conversation by several predetermined alternatives, e.g. by giving another meeting time or place.

The prototype for EMG-based continuous speech recognition is a software package consisting of the recording software and the speech recognition backend engine, both running on a Microsoft Windows PC (Windows XP and Vista have been successfully tested). Besides the software, demonstrating the system requires the recording hardware (amplifier, electrodes, audio headset, and synchronization system) as it is used for recordings with the single-electrode setup described in section 3.1.1. Indeed, enrollment data is recorded in exactly the same way as the EMG-PIT and EMG-UKA corpus data.

The *frontend* software is the *UKA EEG/EMG Studio*, which was already described in section 3.1.1. It not only features a well-designed user interface for data capturing, but also contains a demonstration mode in which it interacts with the JRTk speech recognition engine. Both are used for the prototype, as described below. While the key purpose of the demonstrator is the presentation of silent speech recognition, we also included the sentence-based speech translation engine developed by S. Jou [Jou08] as an optional component.

The *backend* software is a collection of EMG recognition scripts written in TCL, working with the JRTk engine. These scripts are used twice: First, the background system for MLLR adaptation must be trained prior to using the demonstration (this can also be done on a different computer, e.g. a fast server). Second, as soon as enrollment data for MLLR has been recorded, JRTk is used to perform the adaptation and compute updated models.

In the following section, details about the setup of these components is given.

8.3.2 Demo Setup and Presentation

Training of the session-independent background system works exactly as described in section 8.1.1, we do not repeat the description here. Currently, session-independent background systems exist for speakers 2 and 8 of the EMG-UKA corpus, they were trained using six training sessions each consisting of around 70 utterances: For the demonstration, we used slightly enlarged sentence sets, consisting of both a standard 50-sentence corpus as used in our offline experiments, and several additional sentences taken from the "phone call" scenario. Here the number of usable training sentences varies slightly. Otherwise, standard training settings are used.

Assuming that a suitable background system exists, and that the recording apparatus has been prepared for recording data from a demo subject, presenting the prototype now requires two steps:

- Recording of the adaptation sentences and computation of the adapted models.
- Real-time presentation, using either of the two demonstration scenarios described above.

For adaptation, we typically use a set of around 70 sentences, as described above. They are recorded just like any data, i.e. the UKA EEG/EMG Studio is set to recording mode, so that it presents text prompts, allowing the user to collect supervised data. Data is only collected in the audible speaking mode.

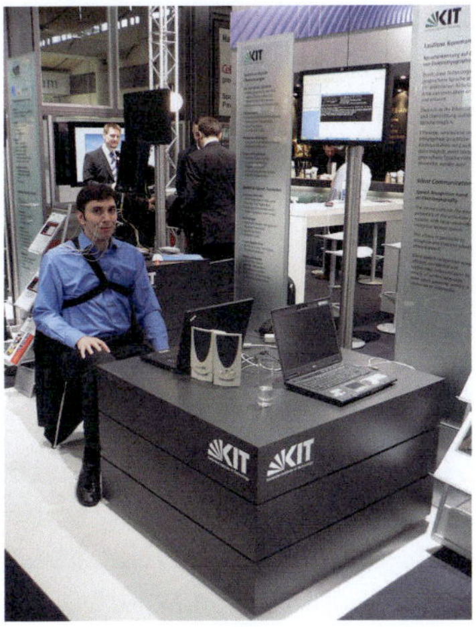

Figure 8.10 – Demonstration of the EMG-based speech recognizer during the CeBIT 2010 fair

When this data has been created, a TCL script comprising the necessary steps for adaptation is started: For the online demonstration, this requires creating a session database and several auxiliary files, computing time-alignments for the adaptation data, and actually collecting statistics and performing the MLLR. Our current main system runs on an Intel Core2 Duo dual-core laptop at 2.53 GHz CPU frequency, here the entire adaptation is performed in 5 – 10 minutes. During the computation of the MLLR, the frontend is not required and may be switched off, however the electrodes should not be detached.

When adapted models have been computed and written to disk, the demonstrator is ready for use. The UKA EEG/EMG Studio frontend is set to demonstration mode, which causes the JRTk backend to start up and enter a waiting loop. The user can now record a single utterance, when the recording is finished, the file is written to disk, and a semaphore file is created to signal the backend that decoding should start. When JRTk has finished decoding the utterance, the resulting text is again written to disk, and another semaphore file is created to make the UKA EEG/EMG Studio read the hypothesis from disk. The hypothesis is then displayed on the screen. On any modern laptop, this process is faster than real-time (for example, processing a 6-second utterance takes 1 – 2 seconds).

8.3.3 Outreach and Feedback

The prototype system has been presented a large number of times, in very different occasions. Demonstrations occured on scientific events, in particular, on the 2009 Interspeech conference in Brighton, UK, where a special session on Silent Speech Interfaces took place. An even greater audience, consisting of both professionals and lay-persons, was reached on the 2010 CeBIT fair (see figure 8.10), which is the largest IT fair worldwide, and on the 2011 fair of the AAAS (American Association for the Advancement of Science). Television appearances of the EMG-based Silent Speech interface include German ZDF and British BBC news.

From the standpoint of the researcher, such demonstrations serve the triple purpose of establishing the practical suitability of the underlying methods, gaining insight into real-life challenges which must be addressed (like the ones mentioned at the beginning of this chapter), and accumulating user feedback (including ideas for usage scenarios of the system). The latter is also a benefit for spectators watching the demonstration, and for the general public: Potential users are made aware of our technology, and by giving feedback, they are able to influence the development and features of the EMG-based speech recognizer.

Chapter 9

Conclusion and Future Work

This final section concludes the thesis and presents directions for future work. We explain in particular how the newly developed algorithms and methods may serve as stepping stones for the ongoing development of the EMG-based speech recognizer, working towards the ultimate goal of applying the system in the real world. This leads to some concrete suggestions for future work, which we give at the very end of this chapter.

We argued in this thesis that EMG-based speech recognition is an active, dynamic field of research, and that the results obtained in this thesis are important stepping stones towards the ambitious goal of practical deployment of the myoelectric Silent Speech interface. We conclude our work by summarizing its central results and contributions and presenting them in a wider context, with a focus on both future reseach efforts and practical usage. We intend to show that the results are part of a wide-scale research effort, which began years ago and certainly is going to be continued in the future.

We point out highlights of the system, but we also raise questions where a desired result has not been achieved. Clearly, a relatively new topic like Silent Speech recognition offers plenty of remaining work for future researchers, so we finally lay out some suggestions and ideas for future work.

9.1 Summary of Thesis Results

The key achievements of this thesis were presented in section 1.5, they structurally follow the central chapters of this work. They were, in order of presentation:

- Introduction of Bundled Phonetic Feature modeling
- Analysis of Silent Speech, and the Spectral Mapping algorithm
- Establishment of the electrode array system
- Session independency and session adaptation
- The online demonstration system

Of these, the first three results are of a theoretical nature, whereas the latter two bridge the gap to practical applications of the technology. All newly developed algorithms yield Word Error Rate (WER) improvements, but what have we gained beyond that?

We believe that many of our results lay important foundations for both practical application and future research. In this section we argue why this is the case; some concrete suggestions for future investigations are presented in section 9.2.

The BDPF Models We first consider our modeling improvements. The BDPF approach described in chapter 5 clearly yields a major accuracy improvement, with over 40% WER reduction. All further experiments in this thesis are heavily based on the BDPF system, in particular, the online demonstration only becomes possible by using BDPF models. We expect this to remain true in the future: At least as long as session-dependent systems remain more robust than session-independent ones, BDPF modeling will be a method of choice.

From a theoretical standpoint, BDPF models allow to use the power of flexible modeling for the small session-dependent EMG corpora, extending the idea of flexible context-dependent speech recognition developed more than 25 years ago. One can additionally argue that BDPF models, due to their automatic, data-driven generation, satisfy a kind of techological optimality criterion: We state that it is always desirable to create features, models, parameters, etc. in a data-driven way, rather than resorting to fixed assumptions, educated guesses or manual parameter optimization. Here classical (in particular, context-independent) phone models represent such a fixed structure with no inbuilt flexibility, and from our initial experiments reported in chapter 4, it becomes clear that they are not optimal (particularly for very small corpora, they tend to incur undertraining). BDPF models are not only better than phone models because they yield improved WERs, but also because they are generated so that they fit the data. (This does by no means preclude that the BDPF tree creation brings its own set of parameters which have to be optimized, e.g. the number of tree leaves: The resulting models are still much more flexible and data-optimized than phone models. Also, the BDPF models behave quite robustly with respect to parameter variations, as described in section 5.2.3).

Altogether, we conclude that the BDPF modeling yielded a major theoretical and practical benefit, and that is forms an indispensable basis for all further experiments.

Silent and Audible Speech This thesis comprises a detailed investigation on the properties of Silent Speech, and on how to deal with it. We consider this a key concern of our work, since processing Silent Speech will be the main purpose of a system used in practice. Silent speech was tackled from three directions (with some additional results on whispered speech):

- Signal-based discrimination of audible and silent speech: How do EMG signals of audible and silent speech differ?
- Influence on the recognizer: How does the recognizer react to discrepancies between speaking modes? Here we used the BDPF tree as a diagnostic tool.
- How to compensate for the different speaking modes: The Spectral Mapping algorithm.

These three points cover many aspects of silent speech and yield important insights: For example, the results on cross-modal testing and cross-modal labeling show that silent speech suffers both from being different from audible speech *and* from being inconsistent. Yet we also proved that it is possible to speak silently and obtain the same signal quality as in audible speech: Speakers 2 and 8 from the EMG-UKA corpus are examples for this.

Still, some research questions remain unresolved. Theoretical aspects include phone-specific investigation of speaking mode differences: while we published some initial results in [JWS10a, JWS10b], a detailed analysis remains missing. Also, while the Spectral Mapping algorithm generates a substantial and significant WER improvement on silent speech, the result is still worse than on corresponding audibly spoken speech. A more versatile signal postprocessing (e.g. by considering phone assignments) might bring some improvement here, and we have laid the foundations for such research. We additionally assume that major improvements will be attained by enhancing the recording procedure: It is probably necessary to give the speaker some kind of *feedback* on the generated EMG signal in order to obtain good silent speech. The initial results we published in [HJWS11] may be a guideline towards developing versatile feedback methods.

Array-based recording system: Versatile EMG processing The initial experiments of this thesis are based on a classical single-electrode setup which has been in use since 2005 [MH05a]. A new recording system based on electrode arrays was developed, expecting advances in signal source decomposition and localization, among other advantages. We have shown that signal source decomposition can be used to build an artifact removal algorithm. Further goals of the EMG array technology remain outstanding; still, our results on Independent Component Analysis show that EMG arrays can be used to extract information which is not available from the single-electrode setup, and that novel algorithms can be based on such information.

Therefore, we expect that EMG array technology will play a central role in future research, and we give some specific suggestions below. Additionally, we state the hypothesis that it will be very hard to achieve substantial gains by varying the signal preprocessing for the *single-electrode* system: at least for audible EMG, the current feature set probably is as good as it gets. We can justify this assumption with some of our side experiments (not reported in this thesis): variations of the feature set, like different frame length or different feature variations, never caused the system to substantially improve or degrade, more complicated features, like frequency features, even caused accuracy deterioration (see e.g. [WJS07, JSW$^+$06]). This might mean that we have reached a level of feature quality which is not easily exceeded.

There is also a theoretical argument: The facial EMG signal is very complex since it consists of superimposed signals from a multitude of sources, yet a small number of single electrodes with rather large surface cannot capture all this complexity: We mostly obtain a representation of local EMG activity, without being able to discern where this activity comes from. Time-domain features, in all their variations, essentially represent the degree of local activity, and the observation that feature variations did not cause major accuracy changes suggests that whatever information can be found in the signal by standard methods is already robustly represented in the currently used time-domain features (including the context stacking).

Session independency, speaker independency, and adaptation We have clearly shown that session-independent systems are not only feasible, but can actually yield similar performance as session-dependent systems, provided that enough training data is available. This is a significant result with a major impact on practical applicability, since session independency means that the system might be pre-trained by a speaker and is then usable without further enrollment: This is an absolute requirement for the vast majority of practical application scenarios.

Our session adaptation methods further extend this line of research: In particular, unsupervised adaptation allows to continuously improve the system based on data collected during usage and thereby bridges the gap between *training data*, which currently still has to be collected in a time-consuming (and boring) process, and *real-life data* accrued during practical system usage, large amounts of which are easily available. On the long run, the Silent Speech recognizer will be trainable with more diverse data than the specific set of sentences which is currently used. Then, unsupervised methods will open the way to using vastly larger amounts of training data than have ever been used before for EMG-based speech recognition.

9.2 Suggestions for Future Work

In the above section, we summarized the main results of this thesis and pointed out results which lay a foundation for future extensions of our research. Here we intend to make some concrete suggestions for future experiments, based on experiences from the work conducted in this thesis. Of course, we do not claim that this list of propositions is complete, or that these methods will actually yield the expected results: Future researchers will answer these questions.

Further integration of EMG array technology A line of research which will certainly play a role in the future is the EMG array technology. We have shown that the high-dimensional array data allows information extraction in a way which is impossible for single-electrode data. Particularly, an artifact detection algorithm based on Independent Component Analysis (ICA) has been developed. In which further ways could one make use of the power of EMG arrays?

Firstly, it will be important to better understand the components and evolution of the EMG signal. This might be tackled as follows.

- Localize EMG signal components: This can be done with a method based on ICA, we presented preliminary results in [Hei13, Chapter 4] and in the conference publication [WHH+13].
- Determine whether certain localized components work well for recognizing certain articulatory movements or phonetic features.

- Determine whether other ICA/source separation approaches (for example, deconvolution [BS95, AS98]) yield better results than out-of-the-box instantaneous ICA.
- In parallel to improving the ICA approach, the raw signal can also be used; in our ongoing work [WSJS14] we use RMS features to detect array repositioning between sessions, and there is indication that there features, although they are simpler than the **TD**n features, are actually very useful for this purpose. Therefore, the EMG feature extraction should be reinvestigated in the light of EMG arrays. From a possible application of RMS features we expect a better visualization and consequently a better understanding of the EMG activity patterns.
- Modeling the temporal evolution: Can one observe EMG components which propagate along the direction of the muscle fibers? Extracting such components might help enormously in decomposing the signal. Here methods of causality (e.g. Granger causality [Gra69]) might be applicable, as they are for EEG signals (see e.g. [BMB$^+$12]).

Further investigations on audible and silent EMG Out of the possible directions with respect to improving the quality of silent speech recognition, we mention three concrete suggestions:

- Phone-based analysis: We reported some initial results on the realization of phones or phonetic features in audible and silent speech in [JWS10a, JWS10b]. A detailed study could build on these results, now with an enlarged corpus and a better baseline accuracy due to improved parameters. The prior results could possibly be enhanced by considering frames larger than the usual 27ms: There are some initial hints that computing the signal energy at the phone level (i.e. with frames of varying size, each as long as a phone) yields a useful signal representation. Such a representation could be used to improve the Spectral Mapping algorithm.
- Integration of the array system: Extracted signal components, as in the ICA experiments, could be examined for differences between audible and silent speech.
- User feedback: In the future, we hope that direct synthesis [TWS09, NJWS11, JWNS12] becomes fast enough to be performed in real-time. In this case, synthesized speech could be played to the user even during recording, yielding accurate feedback and alleviating the loss of articulation preciseness when speaking silently.

User studies So far, all users have been healthy individuals, mostly from the student populations of the cities of Karlsruhe and Pittsburgh. We suggest to plan data recording for speech-disabled persons: This would yield important results not only about practical challenges for deploying the system in this way, but also about the user experience. During the work for this thesis, it became clear that the need for non-acoustic speech processing techniques is high in the speech-disabled community, and that valuable assistance could be gained by opening up the system in such a way.

One prerequisite for this would be that speaker bootstrapping, in particular when only silent speech is used, becomes easier and more robust. An enlarged vocabulary would also be a requirement: Here we hope for positive influence of larger amounts of training data, which can be obtained by using unsupervised methods.

In general, both for speech-handicapped people and for general usage, we state that the time is right for our Silent Speech device to go to the people, rather than stay behind the university walls. We hope that the results of this thesis help to pave the way towards such broad usage of Silent Speech recognition and processing.

Bibliography

[Adi13] Davud Adigüzel. Signalinterpolation für Elektrodenarrays in der EMG-basierten Spracherkennung. Bachelor's thesis, Cognitive Systems Lab, Karlsruhe Institute of Technology, 2013.

[Ale12] Luben Alexandrov. F0-Erkennung bei elektromyographischer Sprachsynthese mit Elektrodenarrays. Bachelor's thesis, Cognitive Systems Lab, Karlsruhe Institute of Technology, 2012.

[AS98] Hagai Attias and Christoph E. Schreiner. Blind Source Separation and Deconvolution: The Dynamic Component Analysis Algorithm. *Neural Computation*, 10:1373–1424, 1998.

[BBdSM86] Lalit R. Bahl, Peter F. Brown, Peter V. de Souza, and Robert L. Mercer. Maximum Mutual Information of Hidden Markov Model Parameters for Speech Recognition. In *Proc. ICASSP*, pages 49 – 52, 1986.

[BdSG+91] Lalit R. Bahl, Peter V. de Souza, Ponani S. Gopalakrishnan, David Nahamoo, and Michael A. Picheny. Decision Trees for Phonological Rules in Continuous Speech. In *Proc. ICASSP*, pages 185 - 188, 1991.

[Bey00] Peter Beyerlein. *Diskriminative Modellkombination in Spracherkennungssystemen mit großem Wortschatz.* Dissertation, RWTH Aachen, 2000.

[Bis07] Christopher M. Bishop. *Pattern Recognition and Machine Learning.* Springer, 2007.

[BMB+12] Adam B. Barrett, Michael Murphy, Marie-Aurelie Bruno, Quentin Noirhomme, Melanie Boly, Steven Laureys, and Anil K. Seth. Granger Causality Analysis of Steady-State Electroencephalographic Signals during Propofol-Induced Anaesthesia. *PLoS ONE*, 7(1):e29072, 2012.

[BNCKG10] Jonathan S. Brumberg, Alfonso Nieto-Castanon, Philip R. Kennedy, and Frank H. Guenther. Brain-computer Interfaces for

Speech Communication. *Speech Communication*, 52:367 – 379, 2010.

[Bro94] Travis Brown. *Historical First Patents: The First United States Patent for Many Everyday Things*. University of Michigan: Scarecrow Press, 1994.

[BS80] Fritz Buchthal and Henning Schmalbruch. Motor Unit of Mammalian Muscle. *Physiological Reviews*, 60:90 – 142, 1980.

[BS95] Anthony J. Bell and Terrence I. Sejnowski. An Information-Maximization Approach to Blind Separation and Blind Deconvolution. *Neural Computation*, 7:1129 – 1159, 1995.

[BS07] Steffen Bickel and Tobias Scheffer. Dirichlet-enhanced Spam Filtering Based on Biased Samples. In B. Schölkopf, J. Platt, and T. Hoffman, editors, *Advances in Neural Information Processing Systems*, pages 161 – 168. MIT Press, 2007.

[BSA00] Armando B. Barreto, Scott D. Scargle, and Malek Adjouadi. A Practical EMG-based Human-computer Interface for Users with Motor Disabilities. *Journal of Rehabilitation Research and Development*, 37(1):53 – 63, 2000.

[BT05] Jeffrey C. Bos and David W. Tack. Speech Input Hardware Investigation for Future Dismounted Soldier Computer Systems. DRCD Toronto CR 2005-064, 2005.

[Car98] Jean-Francois Cardoso. Blind signal separation: Statistical Principles. *Proc. IEEE*, 9(10):2009 – 2025, 1998.

[CC93] Jan P. Clarys and Jan Cabri. Electromyography and the Study of Sports Movements: A Review. *Journal of Sports Sciences*, 11(5):379 – 448, 1993.

[CEHL01] Adrian D. C. Chan, Kevin B. Englehart, Bernie Hudgins, and Dennis F. Lovely. Myoelectric Signals to Augment Speech Recognition. *Medical and Biological Engineering and Computing*, 39:500 – 506, 2001.

[CEHL02] Adrian D. C. Chan, Kevin B. Englehart, Bernie Hudgins, and Dennis F. Lovely. Hidden Markov Model Classification of Myoelectric Signals in Speech. *IEEE Engineering in Medicine and Biology Magazine*, 21(9):143–146, 2002.

[CK79] Peter R. Cavanagh and Paavo V. Komi. Electromechanical Delay in Human Skeletal Muscle under Concentric and Eccentric Contractions. *European Journal of Applied Physiology and Occupational Physiology*, 42(3):159 – 163, 1979.

[Col] OpenStax College. Anatomy & Physiology. Available online: http://cnx.org/content/col11496/1.6. [Last accessed 02-September-2013].

[Com94] Pierre Comon. Independent Component Analysis, a New Concept? *IEEE Transactions on Signal Processing*, 36:287 – 314, 1994.

[CT91] Thomas M. Cover and Joy A. Thomas. *Elements of Information Theory*. J. Wiley, 1991.

[CvdS09] Claudio Castellini and Patrick van der Smagt. Surface EMG in Advanced Hand Prosthetics. *Biological Cybernetics*, 100:35 – 47, 2009.

[Dan80] Gary L. Dannenbring. Perceptual Discrimination of Whispered Phoneme Pairs. *Perceptual and Motor Skills*, 51:979 – 985, 1980.

[DCH$^+$11] Bruce Denby, Jun Cai, Thomas Hueber, Pierre Roussel, Gérard Dreyfus, Lise Crevier-Buchman, Claire Pillot-Loiseau, Gérard Chollet, Sotiris Manitsaris, and Maureen Stone. Towards a Practical Silent Speech Interface Based on Vocal Tract Imaging. In *Proc. 9th International Seminar on Speech Production*, 2011.

[DdRMH$^+$07] Guido Dornhege, José del R. Millán, Thilo Hinterberger, Dennis J. McFarland, and Klaus-Robert Müller, editors. *Toward Brain-Computer Interfacing*. MIT Press, 2007.

[Die08] Maria Dietrich. *The Effects of Stress Reactivity on Extralaryngeal Muscle Tension in Vocally Normal Participants as a Function of Personality*. PhD thesis, University of Pittsburgh, 2008.

[dL79] Carlo J. de Luca. Physiology and Mathematics of Myoelectric Signals. *IEEE Transactions on Biomedical Engineering*, BME-26:313 – 325, 1979.

[dLAW$^+$06] Carlo J. de Luca, Alexander Adam, Robert Wotiz, L. Donald Gilmore, and S. Hamid Nawab. Decomposition of Surface EMG Signals. *Journal of Neurophysiology*, 96:1646 – 1657, 2006.

[dLM88] Carlo J. de Luca and Roberto Merletti. Surface Myoelectric Signal Crosstalk among Muscles of the Leg. *Electroencephalography and Clinical Neurophysiology*, 69:568 – 575, 1988.

[DM04] Arnaud Delorme and Scott Makeig. EEGLAB: An Open Source Toolbox for Analysis of Single-Trial EEG Dynamics including Independent Component Analysis. *Journal of Neuroscience Methods*, 134(1):9–21, 2004.

[DODS06] Bruce Denby, Yacine Oussar, Gérard Dreyfus, and Maureen Stone. Prospects for a Silent Speech Interface Using Ultrasound Imaging. In *Proc. ICASSP*, pages I–365 – I–368, 2006.

[DPH+09] Yunbin Deng, Rupal Patel, James T. Heaton, Glen Colby, L. Donald Gilmore, Joao Cabrera, Serge H. Roy, Carlo J. De Luca, and Geoffrey S. Meltzner. Disordered Speech Recognition Using Acoustic and sEMG Signals. In *Proc. Interspeech*, pages 644 – 647, 2009.

[DS04] Bruce Denby and Maureen Stone. Speech Synthesis from Real Time Ultrasound Images of the Tongue. In *Proc. ICASSP*, pages I–685 – I–688, 2004.

[DSH+10] Bruce Denby, Tanja Schultz, Kiyoshi Honda, Thomas Hueber, and James Gilbert. Silent Speech Interfaces. *Speech Communication*, 52(4):270 – 287, 2010.

[EGJM95] Ellen Eide, Herbert Gish, Philippe Jeanrenaud, and Angela Mielke. Understanding and Improving Speech Recognition Performance Through the Use of Diagnostic Tools. In *Proc. ICASSP*, pages 221 – 224, 1995.

[EHP01] Kevin B. Englehart, Bernie Hudgins, and Philip A. Parker. A Wavelet-Based Continuous Classification Scheme for Multifunction Myoelectric Control. *IEEE Transactions on Biomedical Engineering*, 48:302 – 311, 2001.

[FC86] Alan J. Fridlund and John T. Cacioppo. Guidelines for Human Electromyographic Research. *Psychophysiology*, 23:567 – 589, 1986.

[FCBD+10] Victoria-M. Florescu, Lise Crevier-Buchman, Bruce Denby, Thomas Hueber, Antonia Colazo-Simon, Claire Pillot-Loiseau, Pierre Roussel, Cédric Gendrot, and Sophie Quattrocchi. Silent vs Vocalized Articulation for a Portable Ultrasound-Based Silent Speech Interface. In *Proc. Interspeech*, pages 450 – 453, 2010.

[FEG+08] Michael J. Fagan, Stephen R. Ell, James M. Gilbert, E. Sarrazin, and P. M. Chapman. Development of a (Silent) Speech Recognition System for Patients Following Laryngectomy. *Medical Engineering and Physics*, 30:419 – 425, 2008.

[Fen10] Gu Feng. Initialization Methods for an EMG-based Silent Speech Recognizer. Diploma thesis, Cognitive Systems Lab, Karlsruhe Institute of Technology, 2010.

[FGH+97] Michael Finke, Petra Geutner, Herrmann Hild, Thomas Kemp, Klaus Ries, and Martin Westphal. The Karlsruhe Verbmobil Speech Recognition Engine. In *Proc. ICASSP*, pages I–83 – I–86, 1997.

[FMS+10] David A. Feinberg, Steen Moeller, Stephen M. Smith, Edward Auerbach, Sudhir Ramanna, Matt F. Glasser, Karla Miller, Kamil Ugurbil, and Essa Yacoub. Multiplexed Echo Planar Imaging for Sub-Second Whole Brain FMRI and Fast Diffusion Imaging. *PLoS ONE*, 5:e15710, 12 2010.

[FR97] Michael Finke and Ivica Rogina. Wide Context Acoustic Modeling in Read vs. Spontaneous Speech. In *Proc. ICASSP*, pages 1743 – 1746, 1997.

[Fri89] Jerome H. Friedman. Regularized Discriminant Analysis. *Journal of the American Statistical Association*, 84(405):165 – 175, 1989.

[FTD12] Joao Freitas, Antonio Teixeira, and Miguel Sales Dias. Towards a Silent Speech Interface for Portuguese. In *Proc. Biosignals*, pages 91 – 100, 2012.

[Fuk90] Keinosuke Fukunaga. *Introduction to Statistical Pattern Recognition.* Academic Press, 1990.

[Gal96] Mark J. F. Gales. The Generation and Use of Regression Class Trees for MLLR Adaptation. Technical report, Cambridge University Engineering Department, 1996.

[Gal97] Mark J. F. Gales. Maximum Likelihood Linear Transformations for HMM-Based Speech Recognition. Technical report, Cambridge University Engineering Department, 1997.

[GGT06] Frank H. Guenther, Satrajit S. Ghosh, and Jason A. Tourville. Neural Modeling and Imaging of the Cortical Interactions underlying Syllable Production. *Brain and Language*, 96:280 – 301, 2006.

[GLF+93] John S. Garofolo, Lori F. Lamel, William M. Fisher, Jonathan G. Fiscus, David S. Pallett, Nancy L. Dahlgren, and Victor Zue. TIMIT Acoustic-Phonetic Continuous Speech Corpus. Linguistic Data Consortium, Philadelphia, 1993.

[GOA05] Gonzalo A. García, Ryuhei Okuno, and Kenzo Akazawa. A Decomposition Algorithm for Surface Electrode-Array Electromyogram. *IEEE Engineering In Medicine and Biology Magazine*, 24(4):63 – 72, 2005.

[Gra69] Clive Granger. Investigating Causal Relations by Econometric Models and Cross-spectral Methods. *Econometrica*, 37:424 – 438, 1969.

[GRH+10] James M. Gilbert, Sergey I. Rybchenko, Robin Hofe, Stephen R. Ell, Michael J. Fagan, Roger K. Moore, and Phil Green. Isolated Word Recognition of Silent Speech using Magnetic Implants and Sensors. *Medical Engineering and Physics*, 32:1189 – 1197, 2010.

[Gue95] Frank H. Guenther. Speech Sound Acquisition, Coarticulation, and Rate Effects in a Neural Network Model of Speech Production. *Psychological Review*, 102:594 – 621, 1995.

[GW96] Mark J. F. Gales and Philip C. Woodland. Mean and Variance Adaptation within the MLLR Framework. *Computer Speech and Language*, 10:249 – 264, 1996.

[HAC+07] Thomas Hueber, Guido Aversano, Gérard Chollet, Bruce Denby, Gérard Dreyfus, Yacine Oussar, Pierre Roussel, and Maureen Stone. Eigentongue Feature Extraction for an Ultrasound-based Silent Speech Interface. In *Proc. ICASSP*, pages I–1245 – I–1248, 2007.

[HAH01] Xuedong Huang, Alejandro Acero, and Hsiao-Wuen Hon. *Spoken Language Processing*. Prentice Hall, 2001.

[Ham89] Richard Wesley Hamming. *Digital Filters*. Dover Civil and Mechanical Engineering Series. Dover Publications, 1989.

[HBC+10] Thomas Hueber, Elie-Laurent Benaroya, Gérard Chollet, Bruce Denby, Gérard Dreyfus, and Maureen Stone. Development of a Silent Speech Interface Driven by Ultrasound and Optical Images of the Tongue and Lips. *Speech Communication*, 52:288 – 300, 2010.

[HBC+13] Robin Hofe, Jie Bai, Lam A. Cheah, Stephen R. Ell, James M. Gilbert, Roger K. Moore, and Phil D. Green. Performance of the MVOCA Silent Speech Interface Across Multiple Speakers. In *Proc. Interspeech*, 2013.

[HBD12] Thomas Hueber, Gérard Bailly, and Bruce Denby. Continuous Articulatory-to-Acoustic Mapping using Phone-based Trajectory HMM for a Silent Speech Interface. In *Proc. Interspeech*, 2012.

[HEF+10] Robin Hofe, Stephen R. Ell, Michael J. Fagan, James M. Gilbert, Phil D. Green, Roger K. Moore, and Sergey I. Rybchenko. Evaluation of a Silent Speech Interface Based on Magnetic Sensing. In *Proc. Interspeech*, pages 246 – 249, 2010.

[HEF+13] Robin Hofe, Stephen R. Ell, Michael J. Fagan, James M. Gilbert, Phil D. Green, Roger K. Moore, and Sergey I. Rybchenko. Small-Vocabulary Speech Recognition using a Silent Speech Interface based on Magnetic Sensing. *Speech Communication*, 55:22 – 32, 2013.

[Hei13] Till Heistermann. Decomposition of Multichannel Electromyographic Signals for a Silent Speech Interface. Bachelor's thesis, Cognitive Systems Lab, Karlsruhe Institute of Technology, 2013.

[HFB+06] Johannes Hummel, Michael Figl, Wolfgang Birkfellner, Michael R. Bax, Ramin. Shahidi, Calvin R. Maurer Jr., and Helmar Bergmann. Evaluation Of a New Electromagnetic Tracking System using a Standardized Assessment Protocol. *Physics in Medicine and Biology*, 51:N205 – N210, 2006.

[HGMM03] Masahiko Higashikawa, Jordan R. Green, Christopher A. Moore, and Fred D. Minifie. Lip Kinematics for /p/ and /b/ Production during Whispered and Voiced Speech. *Folia Phoniatrica et Logopaedia*, 55:17 – 27, 2003.

[Him13] Adam Himmelsbach. Rauschunterdrückung durch Quellenseparation in der EMG-basierten Spracherkennung. Bachelor's thesis, Cognitive Systems Lab, Karlsruhe Institute of Technology, 2013.

[HJWS] Till Heistermann, Matthias Janke, Michael Wand, and Tanja Schultz. Spatial Artifact Detection for Multi-Channel EMG-Based Speech Recognition. Biosignals 2014, to appear.

[HJWS11] Christian Herff, Matthias Janke, Michael Wand, and Tanja Schultz. Impact of Different Feedback Mechanisms in EMG-based Speech Recognition. In *Proc. Interspeech*, pages 2213 – 2216, 2011.

[HKSS07] Panikos Heracleous, Tomomi Kaino, Hiroshi Saruwatari, and Kiyohiro Shikano. Unvoiced Speech Recognition Using Tissue-Conductive Acoustic Sensor. *EURASIP Journal on Advances in Signal Processing*, 2007:1–11, 2007.

[HLW03] Han-Pang Huang, Yi-Hung Liu, and Chun-Shin Wong. Automatic EMG Feature Evaluation for Controlling a Prostetic Hand using a

Supervised Feature Mining Method: An Intelligent Approach. In *Proc. ICRA*, pages 220 – 225, 2003.

[HO92] Takaaki Hasegawa and Keiichi Ohtaniakaaki. Oral Image to Voice Converter, Image Input Microphone. In *Proc. IEEE ICCS/ISITA*, pages 617 – 620, 1992.

[Hop06] Philip M. Hopkins. Skeletal Muscle Physiology. *Continuing Education in Anaesthesia, Critical Care & Pain*, 6(1):1–6, 2006.

[HOS+10] Tatsuya Hirahara, Makoto Otani, Shota Shimizu, Tomoki Toda, Keigo Nakamura, Yoshitaka Nakajima, and Kiyohiro Shikano. Silent-speech Enhancement using Body-conducted Vocal-tract Resonance Signals. *Speech Communication*, 52:301 – 313, 2010.

[HOW06] Elizabeth Hume-O'Haire and Stephen Winters. *Distinctive Feature Theory*. John Wiley & Sons, Ltd, 2006.

[HPA+10] Dominic Heger, Felix Putze, Christoph Amma, Thomas Wielatt, Igor Plotkin, Michael Wand, and Tanja Schultz. BiosignalsStudio: A flexible Framework for Biosignal Capturing and Processing. In *Proc. KI*, pages 33 – 39, 2010.

[Hux00] Hugh E. Huxley. Past, Present, and Future Experiments on Muscle. *Philosophical Transactions: Biological Sciences*, 355:539 – 543, 2000.

[HZ04] Ales Holobar and Damjan Zazula. Correlation-based Decomposition of Surface Electromyograms at Low Contraction Forces. *Medical and Biological Engineering and Computing*, 42:487–495, 2004.

[HZ07] Ales Holobar and Damjan Zazula. Gradient convolution kernel compensation applied to surface electromyograms. In Mike E. Davies, Christopher J. James, Samer A. Abdallah, and Mark D. Plumbley, editors, *Independent Component Analysis and Signal Separation*, volume 4666 of *Lecture Notes in Computer Science*, pages 617 – 624. Springer Berlin Heidelberg, 2007.

[Ikk13] Michael Ikkert. Implementierung und Evaluation eines Large Margin Estimation Algorithmus fur HMMs. Diploma thesis, Cognitive Systems Lab, Karlsruhe Institute of Technology, 2013.

[Int99] International Phonetic Association. Handbook of the International Phonetic Association. Cambridge University Press, 1999.

[ITI05] Taisuke Ito, Kazuya Takeda, and Fumitada Itakura. Analysis and Recognition of Whispered Speech. *Speech Communication*, 45:139 – 152, 2005.

[Jan10] Matthias Janke. Spektrale Methoden zur EMG-basierten Erkennung lautloser Sprache. Diploma thesis, Cognitive Systems Lab, Karlsruhe Institute of Technology, 2010.

[JCL97] Biing-Hwang Juang, Wu Chou, and Chin-Hui Lee. Minimum Classification Error Rate Methods for Speech Recognition. *IEEE Transactions on Speech and Audio Processing*, 5(3):257 – 265, 1997.

[JD10] Charles Jorgensen and Sorin Dusan. Speech Interfaces based upon Surface Electromyography. *Speech Communication*, 52:354 – 366, 2010.

[JFH52] Roman Jakobson, Gunnar Fant, and Morris Halle. *Preliminaries to Speech Analysis: the Distinctive Features and their Correlates.* MIT Press, 1952.

[JJWS12] Christian Johner, Matthias Janke, Michael Wand, and Tanja Schultz. Inferring Prosody from Facial Cues for EMG-based Synthesis of Silent Speech. In *Proc. AHFE*, pages 5317 – 5326, 2012.

[JLA03] Charles Jorgensen, Diana D. Lee, and Shane Agabon. Sub Auditory Speech Recognition Based on EMG/EPG Signals. In *Proc. IJCNN*, pages 3128 – 3133, Portland, Oregon, 2003.

[JLL06] Hui Jiang, Xinwei Li, and Chaojun Liu. Large Margin Hidden Markov Models for Speech Recognition. *IEEE Transactions On Audio, Speech, And Language Processing*, 14(5):1584 – 1595, 2006.

[Jou08] Szu-Chen Jou. *Automatic Speech Recognition on Vibrocervigraphic and Electromyographic Signals.* PhD thesis, Language Technologies Institute, Carnegie Mellon University, 2008.

[JSW04] Szu-Chen Jou, Tanja Schultz, and Alex Waibel. Adaptation for Soft Whisper Recognition Using a Throat Microphone. In *Proc. ICSLP*, 2004.

[JSW05] Szu-Chen Jou, Tanja Schultz, and Alex Waibel. Whispery Speech Recognition Using Adapted Articulatory Features. In *Proc. ICASSP*, pages 1009 – 1012, 2005.

[JSW+06] Szu-Chen Jou, Tanja Schultz, Matthias Walliczek, Florian Kraft, and Alex Waibel. Towards Continuous Speech Recognition using Surface Electromyography. In *Proc. Interspeech*, pages 573 – 576, Pittsburgh, PA, Sep 2006.

[JSW07] Szu-Chen Jou, Tanja Schultz, and Alex Waibel. Continuous Electromyographic Speech Recognition with a Multi-Stream Decoding Architecture. In *Proc. ICASSP*, pages IV–401 – IV–404, 2007.

[JWH+14] Matthias Janke, Michael Wand, Till Heistermann, Kishore Prahallad, and Tanja Schultz. Fundamental Frequency Generation for Whisper-To-Audible Speech Conversion. In *Proc. ICASSP*, pages 2598 – 2602, 2014.

[JWNS12] Matthias Janke, Michael Wand, Keigo Nakamura, and Tanja Schultz. Further Investigations on EMG-to-Speech Conversion. In *Proc. ICASSP*, pages 365 – 368, 2012.

[JWS10a] Matthias Janke, Michael Wand, and Tanja Schultz. A Spectral Mapping Method for EMG-based Recognition of Silent Speech. In *Proc. B-INTERFACE*, pages 22 – 31, 2010.

[JWS10b] Matthias Janke, Michael Wand, and Tanja Schultz. Impact of Lack of Acoustic Feedback in EMG-based Silent Speech Recognition. In *Proc. Interspeech*, pages 2686 – 2689, 2010.

[KA98] Nagendra Kumar and Andreas G. Andreou. Heteroscedastic Discriminant Analysis and Reduced Rank HMMs for Improved Speech Recognition. *Speech Communication*, 26:283 – 297, 1998.

[Kar10] Kais Kara. Session-adaptive Speech Recognition based on Surface Electromyography. Student research thesis, Cognitive Systems Lab, Karlsruhe Institute of Technology, 2010.

[KBC99] William F. Katz, Sneha V. Bharadwaj, and Burkhard Carstens. Electromagnetic Articulography Treatment for an Adult With Broca's Aphasia and Apraxia of Speech. *Journal of Speech, Language, and Hearing Research*, 42(6):1355 – 1366, 1999.

[KHM05] Anna Karilainen, Stefan Hansen, and Jörg Müller. Dry and Capacitive Electrodes for Long-Term ECG-Monitoring. In *Proc. SAFE (8th Annual Workshop on Semiconductor Advances for Future Electronics)*, 2005.

[Kir99] Katrin Kirchhoff. *Robust Speech Recognition Using Articulatory Information.* Dissertation, University of Bielefeld, 1999.

[KK02] Karl-Dirk Kammeyer and Kristian Kroschel. *Digitale Signalverarbeitung. Filterung und Spektralanalyse mit MATLAB-Übungen.* Teubner, 2002.

[KKU+02] Evelyne Kohler, Christian Keysers, M. Alessandra Umilta, Leonardo Fogassi, Vittorio Gallese, and Giacomo Rizzolatti. Hearing Sounds, Understanding Actions: Action Representation in Mirror Neurons. *Science*, 297:846 – 848, 2002.

[Kra07] Rüdiger Kramme, editor. *Medizintechnik.* Springer, 2007.

[KS97] Thomas Kemp and Thomas Schaaf. Estimating Confidence Using Word Lattices. In *Proc. Eurospeech*, pages 827 – 830, 1997.

[KWV00] D. L. Keene, S. Whiting, and E. C. Ventureyra. Electrocorticography. *Epileptic Disorders*, 2:57 – 63, 2000.

[Lee88] Kai-Fu Lee. *Large-Vocabulary Speaker-Independent Continuous Speech Recognition: The SPHINX System.* PhD thesis, Carnegie Mellon University, 1988.

[Lee89] Kai-Fu Lee. *Automatic Speech Recognition: The Development of the SPHINX System.* Kluwer Academic Publishers, 1989.

[Lee10] Ki-Seung Lee. Prediction of Acoustic Feature Parameters using Myoelectric Signals. *IEEE Transactions on Biomedical Engineering*, 57:1587 – 1595, 2010.

[LL82] Ronald S. Lefever and Carlo J. De Luca. A Procedure for Decomposing the Myoelectric Signal into its Constituent Action Potentials - Part I: Technique, Theory, and Implementation. *IEEE Transactions on Biomedical Engineering*, 29(3):149 – 157, 1982.

[LLMAM10] Eduardo Lopez-Larraz, Oscar M. Mozos, Javier M. Antelis, and Javier Minguez. Syllable-Based Speech Recognition Using EMG. In *Proc. EMBC*, pages 4699 – 4702, 2010.

[LvDJ+04] Bernd G. Lapatki, Johannes P. van Dijk, Irmtrud E. Jonas, Machiel J. Zwarts, and Dick F. Stegeman. A Thin, Flexible Multi-electrode Grid for High-density Surface EMG. *Journal of Applied Physiology*, 96:327 – 336, 2004.

[LXL82] Ronald S. Lefever, Alan P. Xenakis, and Carlo J. De Luca. A Procedure for Decomposing the Myoelectric Signal Into Its Constituent Action Potentials - Part II: Execution and Test for Accuracy. *IEEE Transactions on Biomedical Engineering*, 29:158 – 164, 1982.

[Mae90] Shinji Maeda. Compensatory Articulation During Speech: Evidence from the Analysis and Synthesis of Vocal Tract Shapes Using an Articulatory Model. In W. J. Hardcastle and A. Marchal, editors, *Speech Production and Speech Modeling*. Kluwer Academic Publishers, 1990.

[MAKG08] Jeffrey D. Meier, Tyson N. Aflalo, Sabine Kastner, and Michael S. A. Graziano. Complex Organization of Human Primary Motor Cortex: A High-Resolution fMRI Study. *Journal of Neurophysiology*, 100:1800 – 1812, 2008.

[May] Chris Mayer. UKA EMG/EEG Studio v2.0.

[MBSY73] H. S. Milner-Brown, R. B. Stein, and R. Yemm. Changes in Firing Rate of Human Motor Units During Linearly Changing Voluntary Contractions. *Journal of Physiology*, 230:371 – 390, 1973.

[MCDH11] Geoffrey S. Meltzner, Glen Colby, Yunbin Deng, and James T. Heaton. Signal Acquisition and Processing Techniques for sEMG based Silent Speech Recognition. In *Proc. EMBC*, pages 4848 – 4851, 2011.

[MDTM89] Michael S. Morse, Susan H. Day, Barbara Trull, and Herman Morse. Use of Myoelectric Signals to Recognize Speech. In *Proc. 11th Annual Conference of the IEEE Engineering in Medicine and Biology Society*, pages 1793 – 1794, 1989.

[Met05] Florian Metze. *Articulatory Features for Conversational Speech Recognition.* Dissertation, University of Karlsruhe, 2005.

[MH05a] Lena Maier-Hein. Speech Recognition Using Surface Electromyography. Diploma thesis, Interactive Systems Labs, University of Karlsruhe, 2005.

[MH05b] Geoffrey S. Meltzner and Robert E. Hillman. Impact of Aberrant Acoustic Properties on the Perception of Sound Quality in Electrolarynx Speech. *Journal of Speech, Language, and Hearing Research Vol.48 766-779 August 2005*, 48:766 – 779, 2005.

[MHMSW05] Lena Maier-Hein, Florian Metze, Tanja Schultz, and Alex Waibel. Session Independent Non-Audible Speech Recognition Using Surface Electromyography. In *Proc. ASRU*, pages 331 – 336, 2005.

[MLM04] Inhyuk Moon, Myoungjoon Lee, and Museong Mun. A novel EMG-based Human-computer Interface for Persons with Disability. In *Proc. ICM*, pages 519–524, 2004.

[MMS85] Tadashi Masuda, Hisao Miyano, and Tsugutake Sadoyama. A Surface Electrode Array for Detecting Action Potential Trains of Single Motor Units. *Electroencephalography and Clinical Neurophysiology*, 60:435 – 443, 1985.

[MP04] Roberto Merletti and Philip A. Parker, editors. *Electromyography - Physiology, Engineering, and Noninvasive Applications.* John Wiley and Sons, Inc., 2004.

[MW02] Florian Metze and Alex Waibel. A Flexible Stream Architecture for ASR Using Articulatory Features. In *Proc. ICSLP*, pages 2133 – 2136, 2002.

[NBHG00] Lawrence C. Ng, Gregory C. Burnett, John F. Holzrichter, and Todd J. Gable. Denoising of Human Speech using Combined Acoustic and EM Sensor Signal Processing. In *Proc. ICASSP*, pages 229 – 232, 2000.

[NJWS11] Keigo Nakamura, Matthias Janke, Michael Wand, and Tanja Schultz. Estimation of Fundamental Frequency from Surface Electromyographic Data: EMG-to-F0. In *Proc. ICASSP*, pages 573 – 576, 2011.

[NKCS06] Yoshitaka Nakajima, Hideki Kashioka, Nick Campbell, and Kiyohiro Shikano. Non-audible Murmur (NAM) Recognition. *IEICE Transactions on Information and Systems*, E89-D:1–8, 2006.

[NKSC03] Yoshitaka Nakajima, Hideki Kashioka, Kiyohiro Shikano, and Nick Campbell. Non-Audible Murmur Recognition Input Interface using Stethoscopic Microphone Attached to the Skin. In *Proc. ICASSP*, pages 127 – 130, 2003.

[NTSS12] Keigo Nakamura, Tomoki Toda, Hiroshi Saruwatari, and Kiyohiro Shikano. Speaking-aid Systems Using GMM-based Voice Conversion for Electrolaryngeal Speech. *Speech Communication*, 54:134 – 146, 2012.

[NWL08] S. Hamid Nawab, Robert P. Wotiz, and Carlo J. De Luca. Decomposition of Indwelling EMG signals. *Journal of Applied Physiology*, 105:700 – 710, 2008.

[Ols72] Harry F. Olson. The Measurement of Loudness. *Audio*, pages 18 – 22, 1972.

[OM82] Mary Joe Osberger and Nancy S. McGarr. Speech Production Characteristics of the Hearing Impaired. In Norman J. Lass, editor, *Speech and Language: Advances in Basic Research and Practice: Volume 8*. Academic Press, London, UK, 1982.

[Osf11] Megan Jo Osfar. Articulation of Whispered Alveolar Consonants. Master's thesis, University of Illinois at Urbana-Champaign, 2011.

[OT] OT Bioelettronica, Torino, Italy. *EMG-USB2 User Manual*.

[PFC06] Robert D. Preuss, Darren R. Fabbri, and Daniel R. Cruthirds. Noise Robust Vocoding at 2400 bps. In *Proc. ICSP*, 2006.

[PH10] Sanjay A. Patil and John H.L. Hansen. The Physiological Microphone (PMIC): A Competitive Alternative for Speaker Assessment in Stress Detection and Speaker Verification. *Speech Communication*, 52:327 – 340, 2010.

[PMEKL02] Roberto D. Pascual-Marqui, M. Esslen, K. Kochi, and D. Lehmann. Functional Imaging with Low Resolution Brain Electromagnetic Tomography (LORETA): A Review. *Methods and Findings in Experimental and Clinical Pharmacology*, 24C:91 – 95, 2002.

[PS12] David Preston and Barbara Shapiro. *Electromyography and Neuromuscular Disorders, 3rd edition.* Saunders, third edition, 2012.

[PWCS09] Anne Porbadnigk, Marek Wester, Jan-P. Calliess, and Tanja Schultz. EEG-based Speech Recognition - Impact of Temporal Effects. In *Proc. Biosignals*, pages 376 – 381, 2009.

[QBM$^+$06] Thomas F. Quatieri, Kevin Brady, Dave Messing, Joseph P. Campbell, William M. Campbell, Michael S. Brandstein, Clifford J. Weinstein, John D. Tardelli, and Paul D. Gatewood. Exploiting Nonacoustic Sensors for Speech Encoding. *IEEE Transactions on Audio, Speech, and Language Processing*, 14:533 – 544, 2006.

[QZH09] Zhihua Qiao, Lan Zhou, and Jianhua Z. Huang. Sparse Linear Discriminant Analysis with Applications to High Dimensional Low Sample Size Data. *International Journal of Applied Mathematics*, 39:48 – 60, 2009.

[Rab89] Lawrence R. Rabiner. A Tutorial on Hidden Markov Models and Selected Applications in Speech Recognition. *Proc. IEEE*, 77(2):257 – 286, February 1989.

[RC04] Giacomo Rizzolatti and Laila Craighero. The Mirror-Neuron System. *Annual Review of Neuroscience*, 27:169 – 192, 2004.

[Ric09] Korin Richmond. Preliminary Inversion Mapping Results with a New EMA Corpus. In *Proc. Interspeech*, pages 2835 – 2838, 2009.

[RKT03] Korin Richmond, Simon King, and Paul Taylor. Modelling the Uncertainty in Recovering Articulation from Acoustics. *Computer Speech and Language*, 17:153 – 172, 2003.

[RRS87] Harald Reucher, Günter Rau, and Jiri Silny. Spatial Filtering of Noninvasive Multielectrode EMG: Part I - Introduction to Measuring Technique and Applications. *IEEE Transactions on Biomedical Engineering*, BME-34:98 – 105, 1987.

[SAH$^+$13] Tanja Schultz, Christoph Amma, Dominic Heger, Felix Putze, and Michael Wand. Biosignale-basierte Mensch-Maschine Schnittstellen. *at – Automatisierungstechnik*, 61(11):760 – 769, 2013.

[Sch72] Martin F. Schwartz. Bilabial Closure Durations for /p/, /b/, and /m/ in Voiced and Whispered Vowel Environments. *Journal of the Acoustical Society of America*, 51:2025 – 2030, 1972.

[Sch00] Tanja Schultz. *Multilinguale Spracherkennung - Kombination akustischer Modelle zur Portierung auf neue Sprachen.* Dissertation, Universität Karlsruhe (TH), 2000.

[Sch06] Rainer Schandry. *Biologische Psychologie.* Beltz Verlag, 2006.

[Sch11] Christopher Schulte. Aufbau eines EMG-basierten Spracherkennungssystems unter Verwendung von Elektrodenarrays. Bachelor's thesis, Cognitive Systems Lab, Karlsruhe Institute of Technology, 2011.

[SG82] George N. Saridis and Thomas P. Gootee. EMG Pattern Analysis and Classification for a Prosthetic Arm. *IEEE Transactions on Biomedical Engineering*, BME-29:403 – 412, 1982.

[SGW+87] Paul W. Schönle, Klaus Gräbe, Peter Wenig, Jörg Höhne, Jörg Schrader, and Bastian Conrad. Electromagnetic Articulography: Use of Alternating Magnetic Fields for Tracking Movements of Multiple Points Inside and Outside the Vocal Tract. *Brain and Language*, 31:26 – 35, 1987.

[SH90] Samuel D. Stearns and Don R. Hush. *Digital Signal Analysis.* Prentice Hall, 1990.

[SKFD10] Kate Saenko, Brian Kulis, Mario Fritz, and Trevor Darrell. Adapting visual category models to new domains. In Kostas Daniilidis, Petros Maragos, and Nikos Paragios, editors, *Computer Vision – ECCV 2010*, volume 6314 of *Lecture Notes in Computer Science*, pages 213 – 226. Springer Berlin Heidelberg, 2010.

[SLH97] Patrick Suppes, Zhong-Lin Lu, and Bing Han. Brain Wave Recognition of Words. *Proceedings of the National Academy of Sciences USA*, 94:14965–14969, December 1997.

[SM10] Thomas Schaaf and Florian Metze. Analysis of Gender Normalization using MLP and VTLN Features. In *Proc. Interspeech*, pages 306 – 309, 2010.

[SMA09] Hamid Reza Sharifzadeh, Ian Vince McLoughlin, and Farzaneh Ahamdi. Voiced Speech from Whispers for Post-Laryngectomised Patients. *IAENG International Journal of Computer Science*, 36:367 – 377, 2009.

[SMFW01] Hagen Soltau, Florian Metze, Christian Fügen, and Alex Waibel. A One-Pass Decoder based on Polymorphic Linguistic Context Assignment. In *Proc. ASRU*, pages 214 – 217, 2001.

[SS07] Fei Sha and Lawrence K. Saul. Large Margin Hidden Markov Models for Automatic Speech Recognition. *Advances in Neural Information Processing Systems*, 19:1249 – 1256, 2007.

[ST85] Noboru Sugie and Koichi Tsunoda. A Speech Prosthesis Employing a Speech Synthesizer – Vowel Discrimination from Perioral Muscle Activities and Vowel Production. *IEEE Transactions on Biomedical Engineering*, 32(7):485 – 490, 1985.

[Str] Randall Stross. The Incredible Talking Machine. *Time Magazine*, June 23, 2010. Available online: `http://www.time.com/time/specials/packages/article/0,28804,1999143_1999210_1999211,00.html` [Last accessed: July 29, 2013].

[SVN37] Stanley S. Stevens, John Volkman, and Edwin B. Newman. A Scale for the Measurement of the Psychological Magnitude Pitch. *Journal of the Acoustical Society of America*, 8:185 – 190, 1937.

[SVS13] Tanja Schultz, Ngoc Thang Vu, and Tim Schlippe. GlobalPhone: A Multilingual Text & Speech Database in 20 Languages. In *Proc. ICASSP*, pages 8126 – 8130, 2013.

[SW96] Daniel L. Swets and John Weng. Using Discriminant Eigenfeatures for Image Retrieval. *IEEE Transactions On Pattern Analysis And Machine Intelligence*, 18(8):831 – 836, 1996.

[SW01] Tanja Schultz and Alex Waibel. Language Independent and Language Adaptive Acoustic Modeling for Speech Recognition. *Speech Communication*, 35:31 – 51, 2001.

[SW10] Tanja Schultz and Michael Wand. Modeling Coarticulation in Large Vocabulary EMG-based Speech Recognition. *Speech Communication*, 52(4):341 – 353, 2010.

[Tar03] John D. Tardelli. Pilot Corpus for Multisensor Speech Processing. Technical report, MIT Lincoln Labs, 2003.

[TBLT10] Viet-Anh Tran, Gérard Bailly, Hélène Loevenbruck, and Tomoki Toda. Improvement to a NAM-captured Whisper-to-Speech System. *Speech Communication*, 52:314 – 326, 2010.

[TSB$^+$00] Ingo R. Titze, Brad H. Story, Gregory C. Burnett, John F. Holzrichter, Lawrence C. Ng, and Wayne A. Lea. Comparison between Electroglottography and Electromagnetic Glottography. *Journal of the Acoustical Society of America*, 107:581 – 588, 2000.

[TWS09] Arthur Toth, Michael Wand, and Tanja Schultz. Synthesizing Speech from Electromyography using Voice Transformation Techniques. In *Proc. Interspeech*, pages 652 – 655, 2009.

[UCL02] UCLA Phonetics Laboratory. Dissection of the Speech Production Mechanism. Technical report, Department of Linguistics, University of California, 2002. Available online: http://www.linguistics.ucla.edu/people/ladefoge/manual.htm.

[UMRR12] Benigno Uria, Iain Murray, Steve Renals, and Korin Richmond. Deep Architectures for Articulatory Inversion. In *Proc. Interspeech*, 2012.

[UNGH00] Naonori Ueda, Ryohei Nakano, Zoubin Ghahramani, and Geoffrey E. Hinton. Split and Merge EM Algorithm for Improving Gaussian Mixture Density Estimates. *Journal of VLSI Signal Processing*, 26:133 – 140, 2000.

[USNIoHa] National Cancer Institute U. S. National Institutes of Health. Seer training modules, head and neck overview. [Online; accessed 03-September-2013].

[USNIoHb] National Cancer Institute U. S. National Institutes of Health. Seer training modules, structure of sceletal muscle. [Online; accessed 23-April-2014].

[VB88] Barry D. Van Veen and Kevin M. Buckley. Beamforming: A Versatile Approach to Spatial Filtering. *IEEE ASSP Magazine*, 5:4 – 24, 1988.

[Wel67] Peter Welch. The Use of Fast Fourier Transform for the Estimation of Power Spectra: A Method Based on Time Averaging over Short, Modified Periodograms. *IEEE Transactions on Audio and Electroacoustics*, 15(2):70–73, Jun 1967.

[Wes06] Marek Wester. Unspoken Speech - Speech Recognition Based On Electroencephalography. Diploma thesis, Interactive Systems Lab, University of Karlsruhe, Germany, 2006.

[WHH+13] Michael Wand, Adam Himmelsbach, Till Heistermann, Matthias Janke, and Tanja Schultz. Artifact Removal Algorithm for an EMG-based Silent Speech Interface. In *Proc. EMBC*, pages 5750 – 5753, 2013.

[WHNT+10] Simon Wiesler, Georg Heigold, Markus Nußbaum-Thom, Ralf Schlüter, and Hermann Ney. A Discriminative Splitting Criterion for Phonetic Decision Trees. In *Proc. Interspeech*, pages 54 – 57, 2010.

[Wie09] Thomas Wielatt. Entwicklung eines Werkzeuges zur Echtzeitvisualisierung von Biosignalen. State Exam Admission Thesis (Zulassungsarbeit), Institut für Sport und Sportwissenschaft Prof. Schwameder, University of Karlsruhe, 2009.

[Wik13a] Wikipedia. Ear — Wikipedia, the free encyclopedia, 2013. [Online; accessed 02-September-2013].

[Wik13b] Wikipedia. Neuron — Wikipedia, the free encyclopedia, 2013. [Online; accessed 02-September-2013].

[Wil66] Robert D. Wilson. A Criticism Of Distinctive Features. *Journal of Linguistics*, 2:195 – 206, 1966.

[WJH+ar] Michael Wand, Matthias Janke, Till Heistermann, Christopher Schulte, Adam Himmelsbach, and Tanja Schultz. Application of Electrode Arrays for Artifact Removal in an Electromyographic Silent Speech Interface. In *Biomedical Engineering Systems and Technologies. International Joint Conference, BIOSTEC 2013, Barcelona, Spain, February 11-14, 2013, Revised Selected Papers*, Communications in Computer and Information Science. Springer Berlin Heidelberg, to appear.

[WJS07] Michael Wand, Szu-Chen Jou, and Tanja Schultz. Wavelet-based Front-End for Electromyographic Speech Recognition. In *Proc. Interspeech*, pages 686 – 689, 2007.

[WJS11] Michael Wand, Matthias Janke, and Tanja Schultz. Investigations on Speaking Mode Discrepancies in EMG-based Speech Recognition. In *Proc. Interspeech*, pages 601 – 604, 2011.

[WJS12] Michael Wand, Matthias Janke, and Tanja Schultz. Decision-Tree based Analysis of Speaking Mode Discrepancies in EMG-based Speech Recognition. In *Proc. Biosignals*, pages 101 – 109, 2012.

[WJS14] Michael Wand, Matthias Janke, and Tanja Schultz. Tackling Speaking Mode Varieties in EMG-based Speech Recognition. *IEEE Transaction on Biomedical Engineering*, to appear, 2014.

[WJTS09] Michael Wand, Szu-Chen Jou, Arthur R. Toth, and Tanja Schultz. Impact of Different Speaking Modes on EMG-based Speech Recognition. In *Proc. Interspeech*, pages 648 – 651, 2009.

[WKJ+06] Matthias Walliczek, Florian Kraft, Szu-Chen Jou, Tanja Schultz, and Alex Waibel. Sub-Word Unit Based Non-Audible Speech Recognition Using Surface Electromyography. In *Proc. Interspeech*, pages 1487 – 1490, 2006.

[WP02] Philip C. Woodland and Daniel Povey. Large Scale Discriminative Training of Hidden Markov Models for Speech Recognition. *Computer Speech and Language*, 16:25 – 47, 2002.

[WS09] Michael Wand and Tanja Schultz. Towards Speaker-Adaptive Speech Recognition Based on Surface Electromyography. In *Proc. Biosignals*, pages 155 – 162, 2009.

[WS10] Michael Wand and Tanja Schultz. Speaker-Adaptive Speech Recognition Based on Surface Electromyography. In Ana Fred, Joaquim Filipe, and Hugo Gamboa, editors, *Biomedical Engineering Systems and Technologies. International Joint Conference, BIOSTEC 2009, Porto, Portugal, January 14-17, 2009, Revised Selected Papers*, volume 52 of *Communications in Computer and Information Science*, pages 271–285. Springer Berlin Heidelberg, 2010.

[WS11a] Michael Wand and Tanja Schultz. Analysis of Phone Confusion in EMG-based Speech Recognition. In *Proc. ICASSP*, pages 757 – 760, 2011.

[WS11b] Michael Wand and Tanja Schultz. Session-independent EMG-based Speech Recognition. In *Proc. Biosignals*, pages 295 – 300, 2011.

[WSJS13] Michael Wand, Christopher Schulte, Matthias Janke, and Tanja Schultz. Array-based Electromyographic Silent Speech Interface. In *Proc. Biosignals*, pages 89 – 96, 2013.

[WSJS14] Michael Wand, Christopher Schulte, Matthias Janke, and Tanja Schultz. Compensation of Recording Position Shifts for a Myoelectric Silent Speech Recognizer. In *Proc. ICASSP*, pages 2113 – 2117, 2014.

[WW83] Bruce B. Winter and John G. Webster. Driven-right-leg Circuit Design. *IEEE Trans. Biomed. Eng.*, BME-30:62 – 66, 1983.

[Yos08] Hirohide Yoshioka. The Role of Tongue Articulation for /s/ and /z/ Production in Whispered Speech. In *Proc. Acoustics*, pages 2335 – 2338, 2008.

[You08] Stephen J. Young. HMMs and Related Speech Recognition Technologies. In Jacob Benesty, M.Mohan Sondhi, and Yiteng(Arden) Huang, editors, *Springer Handbook of Speech Processing*, pages 539–558. Springer, 2008.

[YRT89] Stephen J. Young, N. H. Russell, and J. H. S. Thornton. Token Passing: a Simple Conceptual Model for Connected Speech Recognition Systems. Technical report, Cambridge University Engineering Department, 1989.

[YS03] Hua Yu and Tanja Schultz. Enhanced Tree Clustering with Single Pronunciation Dictionary for Conversational Speech Recognition. In *Proc. Eurospeech*, pages 1869 – 1872, 2003.

[YW00] Hua Yu and Alex Waibel. Streamlining the Front End of a Speech Recognizer. In *Proc. ICSLP*, pages 353 – 356, 2000.

[YZXL13] Bin Yu, Mingxing Zhu, Lisheng Xu, and Guanglin Li. A Pilot Study of High-Density Electromyographic Maps of Muscle Activity in Normal Deglutition. In *Proc. EMBC*, pages 6635 – 6638, 2013.

[ZX11] Hanqing Zhao and Guoqiang Xu. The Research on Surface Electromyography Signal Effective Feature Extraction. In *Proc. of the 6th International Forum on Strategic Technology*, 2011.